Social Structure and Aging

A series of volumes edited by
K. Warner Schaie

AGING, HEALTH BEHAVIORS, AND HEALTH OUTCOMES

Edited by

K. Warner Schaie
The Pennsylvania State University

Dan Blazer
Duke University Medical Center

James S. House
University of Michigan

 LAWRENCE ERLBAUM ASSOCIATES, PUBLISHERS
1992   Hillsdale, New Jersey   Hove and London

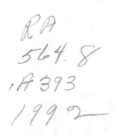

Lawrence Erlbaum Associates, Inc., Publishers
365 Broadway
Hillsdale, New Jersey 07642

Library of Congress Cataloging-in-Publication Data

Aging, health behaviors, and health outcomes / edited by K. Warner
  Schaie, Dan Blazer, James S. House.
        p.   cm. — (Social structure and aging)
    Based on the proceedings of a conference held at the Pa. State
University, Octo. 22–24, 1989 ; sponsored by Penn State Gerontology
Center.
    Includes bibliographical references and index.
    ISBN 0-8058-0780-2
    1. Aged—United States—Health.   2. Afro-American aged—Health.
3. Health behavior.   I. Schaie, K. Warner (Klaus Warner), 1928–
II. Blazer, Dan G. (Dan German), 1944–   . III. House, James S.,
1944–   . IV. Pennsylvania State University. Gerontology Center.
V. Series.
    RA564.8.A393   1992
    362-6—dc20
    DNLM/DLC
    for Library of Congress   91-30972
                                                                    CIP

Printed in the United States of America
10 9 8 7 6 5 4 3 2 1

Contents

Preface

This is the fourth volume in a series on the broad topic of "Social Structure and Aging." It is the edited proceedings of a conference held at the Pennsylvania State University, October, 22–24, 1989. The conference series grew out of a series of planning meetings conducted at the Social Science Research Council by a committee chaired by Matilda White Riley, which called for the systematic exploration of life-course development as a process that is interdependent with social structure and social change. When I assumed the leadership of the Penn State Gerontology Center in 1985, I was pleased to be able to set as one of our goals the implementation of the social structure and aging conference program.

The three previous volumes[1] in this series have dealt with the impact of social structure on aging in psychological processes (Schaie & Schooler, 1989), social structure and aging in cross-cultural perspective (Kertzer & Schaie, 1989), and the impact of social structure in the development of self-efficacy over the life span (Rodin, Schooler, & Schaie, 1990). This volume was designed to highlight the interface between social structures and the behavioral and biological processes of the human aging process specifically as they affect health behaviors and health outcomes in older persons.

---

[1]The three previous volumes are as follows:

Kertzer, D., & Schaie, K. W. (Eds.). (1989). *Age structuring in comparative perspective*. Hillsdale, NJ: Lawrence Erlbaum Associates.

Rodin, J., Schooler, C., & Schaie, K. W. (Eds.). (1990). *Self-directedness: Cause and effects throughout the life course*. Hillsdale, NJ: Lawrence Erlbaum Associates.

Schaie, K. W., & Schooler, C. (Eds.). (1989). *Social structure and aging: Psychological processes*. Hillsdale, NJ: Lawrence Erlbaum Associates.

One of the major concomitants of human aging is the increasing risk of physiological and psychological dysfunctions. Such risk is affected greatly by a variety of social structural variables as well as individual behaviors that mediate favorable or adverse health outcomes. Within this context this volume considers three major questions:

1. What are the effects of social structures and demographic characteristics upon health behaviors?
2. What are the psychosocial influences that affect health outcomes?
3. How do the social structural influences interact with health behaviors to shape the human aging process?

To answer these questions, the editors commissioned chapters that survey the status of social stratification of age and health, both in the general population and among Afro-Americans. Results are reported also from a major epidemiological study, and specific exemplars of the relation between aging, social factors, and health outcomes are provided for the topics of cancer and depression. Each of the primary chapters is followed by comments from experts drawn broadly from the bio-behavioral and social science disciplines. As with previous volumes in this series we think that we have been successful in bridging disciplinary boundaries and we hope that this effort continues our endeavors to permit better communication across disciplines and encourage more effective research on major societal problems related to human aging.

We are grateful for the encouragement and financial support of the conference that led to this volume provided by Anne C. Petersen, Dean of the College of Health and Human Development, and Charles C. Hosler, Vice-President for Research and Graduate Studies of the Pennsylvania State University. We are also grateful to Barbara Impellitteri and Barbara Labinski for handling the conference logistics and to Anna Shuey for coordinating the manuscript preparation. Editorial work for this volume was completed while the senior editor was a Fellow at the Center for Advanced Studies in the Behavioral Sciences, with financial support provided by the John D. and Catherine T. MacArthur Foundation.

K. Warner Schaie

Aging, Health Behaviors, and Health Outcomes:
Goals of the Conference

Dan Blazer
Duke University Medical Center

Despite the emphasis on biological mechanisms and the study of aging and disease during the past decade, an impressive literature has emerged that documents the importance of social factors in disease onset, disease outcomes, health maintenance, and health enhancement (or successful aging). The first goal of the conference participants has been to critically review progress to date across a representative group of studies by prominent investigators in the field. We have learned much during the past decade and we have advanced the field of social behavioral gerontology in the following areas.

First, we have witnessed the publication of seminal articles documenting the role of psychosocial risk factors in prototype community-based, longitudinal studies of risk factors and health outcomes. For example, the importance of behavioral and social factors has been demonstrated in the Framingham Heart Study, the Alameda County Study, and the Evans County Study. Additional studies have been fielded during the past decade, and have solidified the findings from the prototype community studies. These include the Established Population for Epidemiologic Studies of the Elderly (EPESE), the Epidemiologic Catchment Area (ECA) Study, the Michigan Cancer Study, the Edgecomb County Study, and the American Changing Lives Study. Reports from each of these studies were presented during the conference.

Next, we have witnessed the implementation of more sophisticated measures of the independent and control variables. For example, the investigation of stressful life events has been augmented by inquiries into chronic strain. The recognition of the interaction between personality functioning and social ecology is reflected in the study of Type A personality. Social support has emerged as a more proximal variable than previous ecological studies of the social structure and social integration of communities in the exploration of the impact of social factors on health outcomes. Improved delineation of demographic factors, such as the ability to abstract from census data the context of living situations of subjects studied provide new avenues for a contextual analysis. Recent studies have also included relevant control variables, such as health habits, physical functioning, and health services used to ensure the independent role of behavioral and social factors in predicting health outcomes.

We have witnessed a change in the focus of the dependent variables during the past 10 years. For example, studies of "all cause mortality" and functional status have been augmented by studies of hypertension, myocardial infarction, cancer, and major depression as dependent variables. Concentration on more specific disease outcomes has enlightened investigators regarding the relative contribution of different social factors to the web of causation for specific disease entities.

We have available to us and have increasingly used longitudinal data, the only data from which true causal inference can be derived. Although cross-sectional studies remain important first steps and important studies for establishing associates between potential risk factors and health outcomes, the study of large numbers of subjects (representative of large populations) through time, taking advantage of improved field methods, has been a major step in causal analysis. Many questions can now be addressed using longitudinal data sets about which we could only theorize a few years ago.

Finally, we have witnessed the emergence of powerful statistical procedures that enable us to approach cross-sectional and longitudinal data containing many relevant variables simultaneously by use of efficient and interpretable statistical analytic procedures, such as logistic regression and LISREL.

At the same time, we are witnessing an almost exponential advance in the biological sciences. In a society driven by technology, the promise that mechanisms of disease can be identified and simple biological interventions can prevent disease onset and reverse health outcomes is seductively promising. The promises of the biologist have emerged in the midst of a scarcity of resources for science in general. Therefore, social and behavioral scientists are being challenged both by the general public and our biological colleagues to justify the study of social and behavioral factors. We must not close our eyes to this challenge, but rather be prepared to answer it. The format of this conference and the presence of senior investigators in the field of social sciences and social epidemiology provides an opportunity to address a second goal—to answer for ourselves and the scientific community the question "so what?".

"So what" is the true nature and characteristic of the phenomena we study as independent psychosocial risk factors? For example, what is the nature of the variable we label *social support*? Social support is intuitively attractive (like mom and apple pie) but can we say more? Can we be certain that social support is no more than an epiphenomenon, a proxy for personality function or psychological well-being?

"So what" are the mechanisms by which social factors impact disease onset, disease outcomes, health maintenance, and health enhancement? We must transfer clues derived from epidemiologic and sociological surveys to the laboratory, when possible, for more intense study.

"So what" are the public health implications of the findings we report? How do we wish to inform the older adult, the younger adult who anticipates aging, the health-care professional who treats the older adult and the policymaker who allocates scarce resources? In a time of scarce resources, can we convince policymakers of the importance of the social and behavioral factors we have demonstrated to be associated with health outcomes? Science is not best served when it is constantly forced to address "relevant" issues exclusively. Nevertheless, the National Institutes of Health and the National Institute of Mental Health are located within the "Public" Health Service and the public health goals of these agencies that fund most of our research cannot be neglected.

"So what" are the next studies that will advance the field? Large-scale epidemiologic studies? Supplemental studies to ongoing and proposed new large field studies with a more biological orientation? Intensive studies? Laboratory studies? Intervention studies?

We have had an opportunity during this conference to look to the future and address the next generation of studies (or mix of studies) that will best advance an understanding of aging, health behaviors, and health outcomes. This effort represents an opportunity to re-establish our empirical inquiries within a firm theoretical base and to integrate our findings with those of biological scientists and clinicians.

Social Stratification, Age, and Health

James S. House
Ronald C. Kessler
A. Regula Herzog
Richard P. Mero
Ann M. Kinney
Martha J. Breslow
University of Michigan

INTRODUCTION

This chapter integrates and summarizes a line of research developed in somewhat more detail in several other papers (House et al., 1990a, 1990b, 1991). The research derives from an ongoing program project funded by the National Institute on Aging, entitled "Stress, Health and Productive Activity in Middle and Later Life," which seeks to identify psychosocial factors that maintain and enhance health and effective functioning in middle and later life. The work presented here suggests that such psychosocial factors are both macrosocial and microsocial in nature. At the macrosocial level we focus on the system of social stratification in our society. We then try to show how position in the stratification system shapes exposure to microsocial risk factors that are the more proximate determinants of health over the life course.

In this chapter we argue that our society can neither understand nor deal with the related problems of aging and health without coming to grips with what we have come to term the *social stratification of aging and health* (House et al., 1990b, 1991). By this we mean that the way in which health varies by age within and across individuals is heavily influenced by people's socioeconomic status (House et al., 1990a). People of higher socioeconomic status (SES) generally experience high levels of health until quite late in life, whereas people of lower SES are much more likely to manifest significant declines in health by early middle age. Thus, the relation of age to health varies markedly by SES. Furthermore, the relation of SES to health is very different at different points in the life course: SES differences in health are small in early adulthood, increase steadily during middle age and early old age, and then diminish again in advanced old age.

We first suggest theoretically why the relation of age to health should vary across SES levels due mainly to: (a) the differential *exposure* of socioeconomic strata to major psychosocial health-risk factors and (b) the differential *impact* of these risk factors by age. Specifically, we argue that lower SES groups are likely to be more exposed to all psychosocial risk factors, especially in middle and early old age, and the impact of these risk factors is likely to increase with age up through middle age and early old age. Consequently, socioeconomic differentials in health should be greatest in middle age and early old age (when SES differences in exposure to risk factors are greatest and their impact on health is also large) and relatively small in both early adulthood (when SES differences in exposure to risk factors may be sizable but their impact is muted) and advanced old age (when SES differences in exposure to risk factors diminish though their impact remains substantial).

Second, we show empirically in national cross-sectional survey data that the relationship of age to health does vary substantially by SES in the expected way. Further, longitudinal data over 2½ years suggest in a preliminary way that within-individual changes in self-report indicators of health vary by age and socioeconomic status in ways that are consistent with interpreting the cross-sectional data as reflecting a causal impact of socioeconomic status on the way health changes as people age. Third, we show that variations in both the exposure to, and the impact of, psychosocial risk factors across SES and age are generally as we expect if these factors are to explain the observed social stratification of aging and health. Fourth, we demonstrate that adjusting for this pattern of differential exposure to, and impact of, psychosocial risk factors can largely account for or explain the observed social stratification of aging and health. Finally, we discuss the implications of these ideas and data for what we and others take to be the fundamental agenda for research and policy on aging and health; that is, to understand what factors determine the relation of age to morbidity, functional capacity, and mortality, and the extent to which these factors make it possible to postpone morbidity and functional limitations into an increasingly brief final phase of the finite, although not perhaps fixed, human life span (*Gerontologica Perspecta,* 1987).

WHY SHOULD THE PROCESS OF AGING AND HEALTH BE STRATIFIED SOCIOECONOMICALLY?

Human life expectancy has increased more in the last century than in all prior history (Preston, 1977). At the same time, two other aspects of the biology and sociology of human health and aging have remained remarkably invariant. First, the maximal human life span has not increased commensurately with life expectancy, if at all (Fries, 1980). Second, socioeconomic differentials in mortality, disability, and morbidity have remained remarkably persistent in the United States and other developed countries (Fingerhut, Wilson, & Feldheim, 1980; Kitigawa & Hauser, 1973; Marmot, Kogevinas, & Elston, 1987; Syme & Berkman, 1976; Williams, 1990). Each of these persisting verities raises important scientific and policy issues regarding human aging and health, yet socioeconomic status (or indicators of it such as education, occupation, or income) is not even considered in recent overviews of government statistics on aging and health (e.g., Brody, Brock, & Williams, 1987; National Center for Health Statistics, 1987), and is treated only cursorily in major reviews of the literature on aging and health (e.g., Shanas & Maddox, 1985).

The dramatic increase of life expectancy in the face of a finite human life span (of about 85 to 90 years on average) has suggested both utopian and dystopian scenarios for the future. The utopian scenario argues that continuing improvements in health and life expectancy will increasingly postpone or "compress" morbidity and disability into a relatively brief period at the end of the life span, thus improving the quality of life and perhaps even reducing the need for medical care (Fries, 1980). The dystopian scenario suggests that recent and future gains in life expectancy largely add years to life in which people are chronically ill and disabled, and thus high consumers of health care (Gruenberg, 1977; Manton, 1982; Schneider & Brody, 1983; Verbrugge, 1984).

Which scenario proves correct depends on the extent to which currently observed declines in physical and psychological functioning with age are intrinsically linked to the biological process of aging (and thus, not readily preventable or postponable), or are determined by factors extrinsic to that process (and hence more preventable or postponable). Such extrinsic factors are increasingly likely to be social, psychological, and behavioral in nature because morbidity, disability, and mortality in middle and older age are largely a function of chronic diseases, the etiology and course of which are increasingly determined by social, psychological, and behavioral factors (Rowe & Kahn, 1987).

Both theory and data now indicate that SES is a major determinant of the degree to which mortality, morbidity, and disability are postponed into the last phase of the finite human life span (House et al., 1990a). That is, people in the upper socioeconomic strata increasingly approximate the utopian scenario of longer life and better health, with not only mortality but also morbidity and disability or functional limitations generally postponed to quite late in life. In contrast, people in the lower socioeconomic strata experience significant levels of mortality, morbidity, and disability beginning relatively early in mid-life. Thus, with increasing age, levels of health become increasingly differentiated by SES, until the final period of the normal human life span when both biological and social forces tend again to reduce socioeconomic differences.

We believe this social stratification of aging and health is produced by social and biological mechanisms that determine both exposure to, and the impact of, a set of psychosocial variables that have been increasingly recognized as major determinants or risk factors for chronic disease mortality, morbidity, and disability. These include: (a) health behaviors such as smoking and im-moderate eating (leading to under or overweight) or drinking (Berkman & Bres-low, 1983); (b) lack of social relationships and supports (House, Landis, & Um-berson, 1988); (c) lack of what is variously termed *self-efficacy, self-directedness, competence, mastery,* or *control* (Rodin, 1986; Rodin, Schooler, & Schaie, 1990; Rowe & Kahn, 1987); and (d) chronic and acute stress (House, 1987; Pearlin, Lieberman, Menaghan, & Mullan, 1981; Theorell, 1982; Thoits, 1983). A small but growing body of theory and evidence suggests that all of these risk factors are more prevalent in lower socioeconomic groups (Williams, 1990). For some variables this may become increasingly true with age as SES becomes more fixed and more cumulative in its effects through middle and early old age. These differences may, however, be muted in later old age. In recent decades our society has *directly* invested more heavily in improving the social, economic, and health-care status of the older population, as compared to children and younger adults (Duncan & Smith, 1989; Preston, 1984). These social welfare policies, as well as other changes in the biological, social, and psychological status of people as they age may serve to attenuate socioeconomic differences in exposure to psychosocial risk factors in older age.

Additionally, there is reason to believe that the *impact* of many or most of these psychosocial risk factors increases with age, at least until early old age (House & Robbins, 1983). Biologically, people become more vulnerable to a wide range of diseases with age. Socially and psychologically, issues like the maintenance and loss of social relationships and supports or of self-efficacy and control may become more problematic and hence more consequential in older age (e.g., House & Robbins, 1983; Rodin, 1986).

In summary, scattered but growing bodies of theory and data suggest that the process by which health changes with age may be importantly stratified by SES. On average, we should see the largest socioeconomic differentials in health in middle and early old age because these age groups are most likely to be characterized by both sizable SES differentials in exposure to risk factors and substantial impact of the risk factors. In contrast, in early adulthood, SES differences in exposure may be sizable but their health impact is muted, whereas in later old age SES differences in exposure become somewhat muted even if their impact remains strong. Let us now consider how well available data ac-cord with these expectations.

METHODS

Data Sources

Our principal data source is an ongoing longitudinal survey, entitled Ameri-cans' Changing Lives (or ACL), carried out by the Survey Research Center of the University of Michigan on a multi-stage, stratified, area probability sam-ple of noninstitutionalized persons 25 years of age or older and living in the

coterminous United States, with oversampling of Blacks and persons age 60 + .
Initial face-to-face interviews (known as ACL 1) lasting 86 minutes on average were carried out in mid-1986 in the homes of 3,617 respondents, reflecting a response rate of 67% of all designated sample respondents (and 70%
of designated households and of designated individuals who spoke English or
Spanish and were physically and mentally capable of being interviewed). A
total of 2,867, or over 83% of the surviving 1986 respondents participated in
an 83-minute follow-up interview (known as ACL 2) in early 1989, and constitute our current longitudinal sample with about 2.5 years between waves.
Some parallel analyses were conducted for persons age 25 and over in the 1985
National Health Interview Survey (or NHIS), also a multi-stage, stratified,
area probability sample of the total noninstitutionalized U.S. population
(NCHS, 1986). Data are weighted in all analyses to adjust for variations in
selection probabilities and response rates, and all significance tests in the ACL
data are adjusted for sample clustering and weighting (see House et al., 1990a,
1990b, 1991 for details).

Health Measures

Our analyses of the ACL data predicted three self-report indicators of physical
health: (a) a count of 10 major *chronic conditions* experienced in the previous
year (i.e., arthritis/rheumatism, lung disease, hypertension, heart attack or
heart trouble, diabetes, cancer/malignant tumor, foot problems, stroke, fractures or broken bones, and loss of urine beyond one's control); (b) an index
of *functional status,* with the lowest score of 1 indicating confinement to a bed
or chair and the highest score of 4 indicating ability to do heavy work around
the house without difficulty; and (c) a single item self-rating of the extent of
health-related *limitation of daily activities,* where the lowest value of 1 indicates
that a person's daily activities are limited "a great deal" by health or health-
related problems and the highest value of 5 indicates that the person's daily
activities are limited "not at all" by health-related problems.

Socioeconomic Status Measure

Although we generally do not favor the use of indices of SES, we have chosen
to use one here primarily for purposes of economy and feasibility in analyzing
and presenting results. Extensive additional analyses suggest that the two components of the index—education and income—are, along with age, the most
important sociodemographic predictors of morbidity and functional limitations.
Further, the effects of education and income are generally similar, and the SES
index used here effectively captures most of the information contained in the
separate education and income measures and any interactions among them

(see House et al., 1990a, 1990b, 1991). The health impact of education is generally linear and monotonic, whereas for income there are rapidly diminishing
differences in health above the $20,000 level. Thus, we arrive at four levels
of socioeconomic status: (a) *upper* SES, defined as 16 + years of education *and*
income $\geq$ $20,000 ($n$ = 606 at ACL 1); (b) *upper middle* SES, defined as 12–15
years of education *and* income $\geq$ $20,000 ($n$ = 1,346); (c) *lower middle* SES,
defined as either 0–11 years of education *or* income < $20,000 *but not both* ($n$
= 964); and (d) *lower* SES, defined as both 0–11 years of education *and* income < $20,000 ($n$ = 701).

The SES variable is *not* considered to measure prestige or anything other
than the combination of current income and education. We recognize that the
same level of education or income can mean different things in different age
groups, but the rank ordering of levels remains invariant across age groups,
and it is the difference between SES ranks that is of most interest in our and
other analyses of socioeconomic differentials in health.

Education is clearly temporally and hence probably causally prior to health at
age 25 and up; income may be more reciprocally related to health. The essential findings reported here, however, hold if only education is considered. Income partially mediates the effects of education, but has substantial additive
effects and interacts significantly with age even net of the parallel effects of
education. Further, there is good reason to believe that much of the association between income and health reflects a causal impact of income on health
(Fox, Goldblatt, & Jones, 1985; Mechanic, 1968; Wilkinson, 1986). Thus, we
feel it is appropriate to examine the health effects of both income and education in our cross-sectional analyses.

NHIS Measures and Analyses of Sociodemographics and Health

We have replicated the ACL findings on the relationship between age and physical health across levels of socioeconomic status using data from the 1985 National Health Interview Survey (NCHS, 1986). The age and SES variables
used here are the same as in ACL and the NHIS contains similar measures
of chronic conditions and activity limitations (see House et al., 1990a for details on these measures).

Psychosocial Risk Factors

Finally, we return to the ACL data to examine potential explanations of observed differences in health by age and SES in terms of psychosocial risk factors. We consider measures of four types of potential psychosocial explanatory
variables, as indicated in Table 1.1:

TABLE 1.1
Psychosocial Risk Factor Variables

Variables	Scoring
1. *Health Behaviors*	
a. Cigarette smoking	Current smoker = 1; nonsmoker = 0
b. Relative weight	Moderate = 1; over *or* under = 0
c. Alcoholic drinking	Moderate = 1; Heavy *or* none = 0
2. *Social Relationships and Supports*	
a. Marital status	Dummy variable classification
b. Frequency of formal social contacts	Standardized index of two items
c. Frequency of informal social contacts	Standardized index of two items
d. Perceived support from friends and relations	Standardized index of four items
3. *Acute and Chronic Stress*	
a. Negative lifetime events	Number (out of four)
b. Negative events in last 3 years	Number (out of six)
c. Chronic financial stress	Standardized index of three items
4. *Self-Efficacy*	Standardized index of six items

1. *health behaviors* (current smoking vs. nonsmoking; moderate relative weight vs. clear over- or under-weight and moderate drinking vs. non- or heavy-drinking);

2. *social relationships and supports* (marital status, and indices of formal and informal social contacts or integration and of perceived support from friends and relatives);

3. *acute and chronic stress* (lifetime frequency of potentially stressful events, frequency of potentially stressful recent events in the last three years, and an index of chronic financial stress); and

4. *self-efficacy,* an index combining three items from Rosenberg's (1965) self-esteem scale and three items from Pearlin et al.'s (1981) mastery scale (see House et al., 1990b, 1991 for further details on these measures).

Analyses

All analyses derive from OLS regressions of the health measures on SES, either alone, or with adjustments for race and sex, and psychosocial risk factors and their interactions with age as described more fully later. Results are presented in terms of unadjusted or adjusted means by age and SES or regression coefficients and equations.

RESULTS

SES Variation in the Relation of Age to Health

ACL Cross-Sectional Analyses.   Figures 1.1 to 1.3 (adapted from House et al., 1990a) display graphically a striking pattern of differences in the relation of age to health across levels of socioeconomic status in the 1986 ACL cross-section. Figure 1.1 shows that significant numbers of chronic conditions begin to manifest themselves in the American population by middle adulthood, but the relation of the prevalence of chronic conditions to age varies markedly by so-

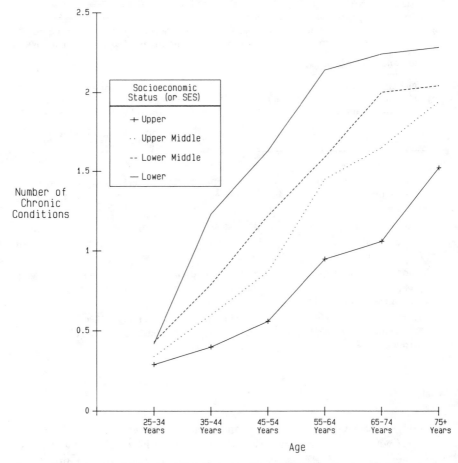

FIG. 1.1.   Age by number of chronic conditions within levels of socioeconomic status (see text for definition of SES levels in terms of education and income). *Source:* House et al. (1990b). 1986 Americans' Changing Lives Interview Survey data, *n* = 3,617 (adapted from House et al., 1990a).

cioeconomic status. In early adulthood (ages 25–34), there are no significant ($p \leq .01$) socioeconomic differences in prevalence of chronic conditions—all socioeconomic groups having an average level of less than 0.5 conditions per person. However, marked socioeconomic disparities emerge by early middle age (35–44) and continue to increase in magnitude up to the time of late middle age/early old age (55–74), and then begin to converge. We have replicated the results shown in Fig. 1.1 for each condition and for three subsets of chronic conditions (a) "potentially life-threatening" (cancer, heart attack/trouble, stroke), (b) "serious chronic" (arthritis, lung disease, hypertension, diabetes, urinary incontinence), and (c) "other" (fractures and foot problems). The pattern of results in Fig. 1.1 is generally replicated in each case, indicating that these results are not unique to, or an artifact of, particular more or less serious health problems.

In Fig. 1.1, the lowest socioeconomic stratum manifests a prevalence of chronic conditions at ages 35–44 that is not seen in the highest socioeconomic stratum until after age 75, and the socioeconomic differential in level of chronic conditions does not begin to converge until after age 75. Considerable postponement of morbidity is evident in the highest socioeconomic group, where the mean prevalence of the 10 chronic conditions included in our measures remains below 0.5 until age 54, and below 1.0 until age 75, when it begins a more marked increase. The other groups do not manifest significant postponement of morbidity into later life, but differ in the rate of the relatively linear increase in chronic conditions with age.

Figures 1.2 and 1.3 show the results for two indicators of functional health. Declines in functional capacity tend generally to be more postponed or compressed into the later stages of life, compared to increases in morbidity. Again, however, it is the pattern of differences by SES in the relation of age to health that is striking: Socioeconomic differences are virtually nonexistent at ages 25–34, then increase markedly through ages 55–64, then begin to converge. For the high socioeconomic group, it is not until age 75 and over that the prevalence of substantially diminished functional capacity is evident. The upper middle socioeconomic group has an almost identical pattern to the high socioeconomic group in both Fig. 1.2 and 1.3, except for a nonmonotonic drop in the 55- to 64-year-old age group. In contrast, the lower socioeconomic groups manifest an essentially linear decline in functional health, with the lowest socioeconomic group having dropped more than a full point on each measure prior to age 65, levels not reached in the higher socioeconomic groups until after age 75. Thus, the upper socioeconomic groups manifest substantial postponement or compression of functional limitations into the last years of life, but the lower socioeconomic groups experience significant functional limitations quite early.

The evidence for postponement of morbidity and disability in the highest SES strata and the absence thereof in the lower SES strata is even more marked

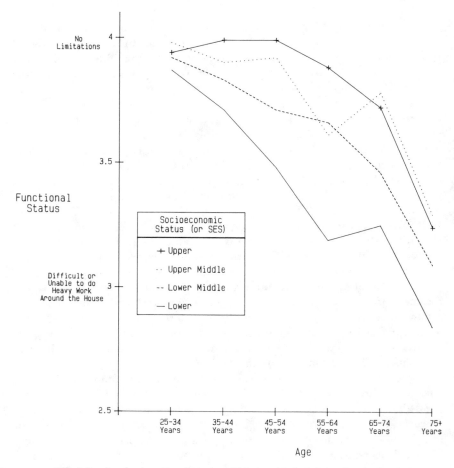

FIG. 1.2. Age by functional status within levels of socioeconomic status (see text for definition of SES levels in terms of education and income). *Source:* House et al. (1990b). 1986 Americans' Changing Lives Interview Survey data, *n* = 3,617 (adapted from House et al., 1990a).

in terms of severe levels of morbidity or functional limitations. Across all SES groups, only 0.5%–1.4% of persons report three or more chronic conditions at ages 25–34. In the highest SES group, the prevalence of this level of multiple morbidity never exceeds 16% even at ages 75 +, whereas 12% of the lowest SES strata report three or more chronic conditions at ages 35–44, rising to 26% by ages 45–54, and 39% prior to age 65. Similarly, the percentage of persons who are unable to walk a few blocks or climb a few flights of stairs without difficulty is 3% or less across all SES groups at ages 25–34. In the upper SES stratum, this percentage rises to only 5% at 65–74 and 9.3% at ages 75 +; but in the lowest SES stratum 12% of persons ages 35–44 report this

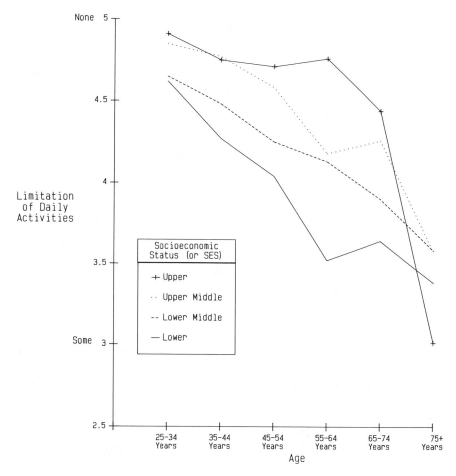

FIG. 1.3. Age by degree of limitation of daily activities within levels of socioeconomic status (see text for definition of SES levels in terms of education and income). *Source:* House et al. (1990b). 1986 Americans' Changing Lives Interview Survey data, *n* = 3,617 (adapted from House et al., 1990a).

level of functional limitation, rising to 29% at ages 55–64 and over 40% at ages 75 +.

1985 NHIS Replication.   Before beginning to interpret the pattern of results in Fig. 1.1 to 1.3, a pattern we had not seen reported elsewhere, we sought to replicate the analyses of the 1986 ACL data in the 1985 National Health Interview Survey (NHIS) which included very similar measures of reports of chronic conditions and limitation of daily activities. The results, presented in Fig. 1.4 and 1.5 (from House et al., 1990a), are strikingly similar to those in

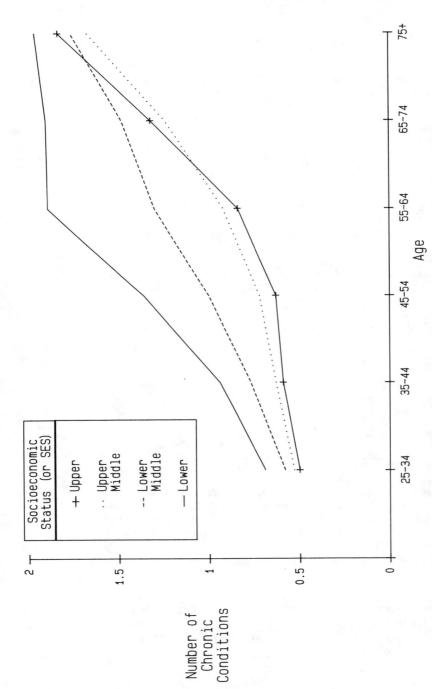

FIG. 1.4. Age by number of chronic health conditions, within one of six health domains and within levels of socioeconomic status (see text for definition of SES levels in terms of education and income). *Source:* House et al. (1990a). 1985 National Health Interview Survey data, *n* = 55,690

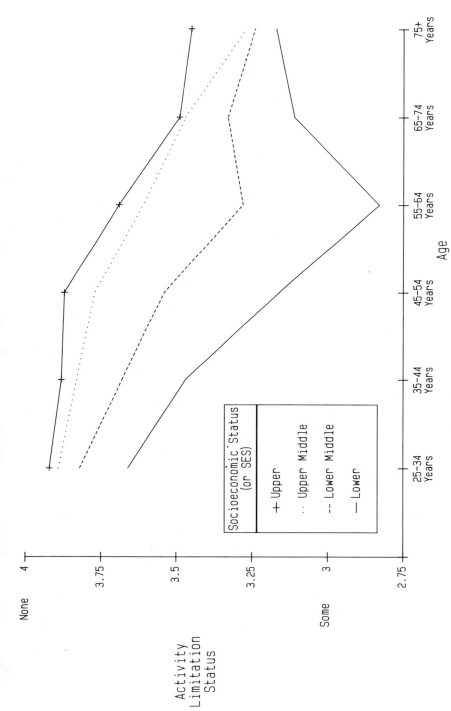

FIG. 1.5. Age by activity limitation status within levels of socioeconomic status (see text for definition of SES levels in terms of education and income). *Source:* House et al. (1990a). 1985 National Health Interview Survey data, *n* = 55,690.

Fig. 1.1 and 1.3, except that the upper middle socioeconomic group is more similar to the highest group and there is perhaps a little more convergence across socioeconomic groups at ages 75 + . Again, we see the two lower socioeconomic strata manifesting in middle age (45–64) levels of chronic conditions and of limitation of functional capacity that are not evident in the higher socioeconomic groups until after age 75, if then (see House et al., 1990a for further details).

In both the ACL and the NHIS data we have checked further for possible higher-order interactions among gender, race, age, and SES. Statistical tests are difficult because of the low numbers of older Blacks of higher SES, but examination of figures such as Fig. 1.1 to 1.5 within gender and race groups (i.e., Black males, Black females, non-Black males, and non-Black females) suggests that the interactions of age with SES do not vary notably by gender or race or a combination thereof.

ACL 1–ACL 2 Longitudinal Analysis.   We interpret the cross-sectional data reported here as indicating that, compared to higher SES persons, the health of individuals in lower SES groups declines more rapidly as they age, especially during middle or early old age. Long-term longitudinal data are ultimately necessary to establish more firmly a causal impact of SES on the way in which health declines with age, as well as to test fully the explanations in terms of psychosocial risk factors that we explore cross-sectionally later. We know of no data set adequate to this task at this point, but can report data from initial analyses of our 1986–1989 longitudinal panel. Because we have only 2.5 years between waves, the degree of change in the health measures is necessarily small (a mean change of .15–.30 on indices with ranges of 1–4, 1–5, and 1–10), with chronic conditions being most stable, reported limitation in daily activities changing the most, and functional health in between. Thus, we cannot yet do analyses in the longitudinal data that fully parallel our cross-sectional analyses. We have, however, predicted change over time in each of our health outcomes between 1986 and 1989 as a function of SES, race, gender, and psychosocial risk factors. These analyses have been done within each of four age groups representing four meaningful life course stages: early adulthood (25–34 in 1986), early middle age (35–54), later middle age or early old age (55–74) and advanced old age (75 +).

If our cross-sectional results reflect a deleterious causal impact of SES on health as individuals age, which is most pronounced in middle age and early old age and explained by differential exposure and impact of psychosocial risk factors, then the following should be true in the longitudinal data:

1. significant declines in health between 1986 and 1989 should be concentrated in lower socioeconomic strata, and within those strata be greatest in middle age and early old age;

2. psychosocial risk factors in 1986 should predict health changes from 1986 to 1989 in expected ways; and

3. controlling for the psychosocial risk factors should, at least partially, explain away the deleterious effects of low 1986 SES on changes in health from 1986 to 1989, again especially in middle age and early old age.

We have tested these expectations by regressing 1989 health measures, within the four age groups just mentioned, first on their 1986 counterparts and race, gender, and SES, and then on these same variables plus psychosocial risk factors. Given the preliminary nature of the test, the results accord surprisingly well with our expectations. The best confirmation occurs for perceived limitation of daily activities, the health measure that shows the most change between 1986 and 1989. At all age levels the lowest socioeconomic stratum shows the greatest deterioration on this measure, but those declines are greatest in the age ranges of 35–54 and 55–74, and there are also sizable declines in these age ranges for the lower middle socioeconomic group as well. In contrast, the two upper socioeconomic strata show no significant change in limitation of daily activities. Finally, the 1986 levels of psychosocial risk factor variables in Table 1.1 generally predict changes in limitation of daily activities as expected, and partially explain the longitudinal effects of SES. Results for the functional status index, which declines somewhat less from 1986 to 1989, are similar to, but less strong and consistent than, the results for limitation of daily activities. Changes in number of chronic conditions are slight and largely random (see House et al., 1990b for details). Longer periods of longitudinal follow-up are necessary to confirm that the cross-sectional results in Fig. 1.1 to 1.5 reflect within-individual changes with aging, but these preliminary results are consistent with that interpretation.

Differential Exposure to Psychosocial Risk Factors as an Explanation. We now turn to the 1986 ACL cross-section to estimate how well patterns of *exposure* to social, psychological, and behavioral risk factors can explain the social stratification of aging and health evident in Fig. 1.1 to 1.3. Our data show that lower SES individuals are disadvantaged on every risk factor we consider. For several psychosocial risk factors—moderate drinking, marital status, informal social integration, and financial chronic stress—the lower SES disadvantage is invariant across age groups, although the relation of age to these risk factors varies. Rates of moderate drinking are relatively constant across age, as are rates of being married until late in life; levels of informal social integration decline into middle age, then rise in older age groups; and levels of chronic financial stress decline with age.

Most of the risk factors, however, show a pattern of modest to sizable lower SES disadvantage in early adulthood, which increases during middle age, and then diminishes during later middle and old age, with the extent and timing of that convergence varying across risk factors. Figures 1.6 and 1.7 show the

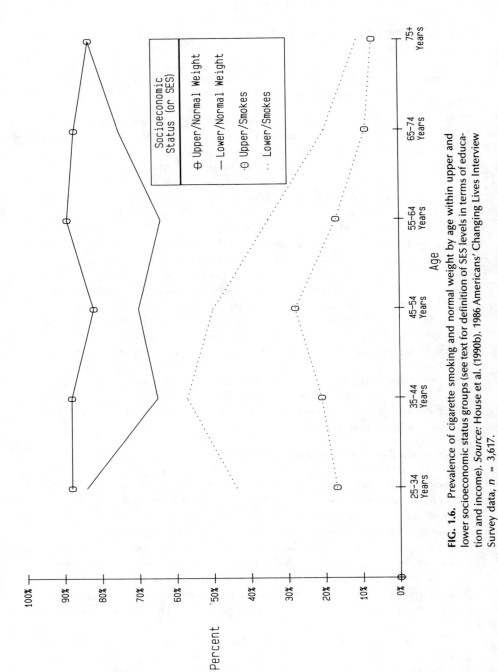

FIG. 1.6. Prevalence of cigarette smoking and normal weight by age within upper and lower socioeconomic status groups (see text for definition of SES levels in terms of education and income). *Source:* House et al. (1990b). 1986 Americans' Changing Lives Interview Survey data, *n* = 3,617.

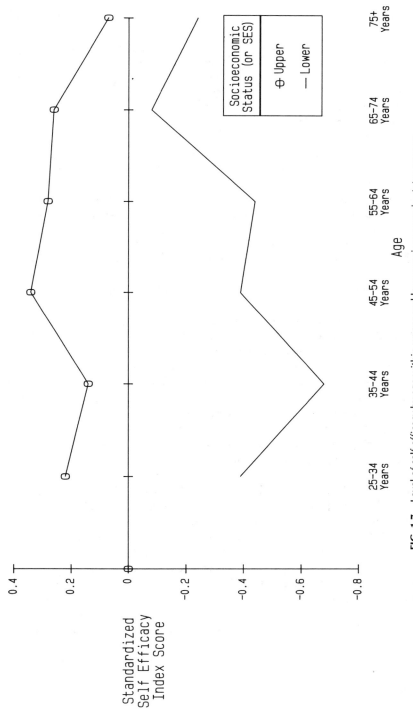

FIG. 1.7. Level of self-efficacy by age within upper and lower socioeconomic status groups (see text for definition of SES levels in terms of education and income). *Source:* House et al. (1990b). 1986 Americans' Changing Lives Interview Survey data, *n* = 3,617.

precise nature of these patterns on several variables for the two extreme SES groups: smoking and relative weight in Fig. 1.6 and self-efficacy in Fig. 1.7. Formal social integration, perceived support from friends and relatives, and recent and lifetime negative events all show similar patterns (not graphed here, but see House et al., 1990b).

Overall, we see a consistent pattern of lower SES disadvantage in exposure to a wide range of social, psychological, and behavioral risk factors, with this disadvantage on average being sizable even at age 25–34, growing larger into middle age and then beginning to decline so that differences on many risk factors become small or nonexistent by early old age (ages 65 +). These differentials in exposure to psychosocial risk factors should contribute significantly to explaining the observed social stratification of aging and health. Risk factor exposure alone is likely to explain a great deal of the SES differences at younger ages, where the differences in exposure are largest, but to account for increasingly less of the SES differentials in health in later middle and early old age where the differences in exposure diminish in many risk factors.

We have empirically tested these inferences regarding the effects of exposure in the 1986 ACL cross-section by estimating regressions of the health variables on dummy variable classifications representing race, gender, the interaction of age and SES, and the dummy and continuous variables representing the 11 risk factors. These analyses show that all of the psychosocial risk factors are related to health as expected—better health habits, higher levels of social relationships and supports, lower levels of chronic and acute stress, and greater self-efficacy are all associated with lower levels of morbidity and functional limitations. The effects of moderate weight, self-efficacy, and chronic and acute stress are generally the strongest, with the effects of smoking, drinking, and social relationships being weaker, both absolutely and relative to the other variables and expectations derived from prior literature. Nevertheless, and recognizing the limitation of cross-sectional data, these psychosocial variables are consequential risk factors for health, together adding about 6% to the explained variance in the dependent variables over and above that explained by age, SES, race, and gender (see House et al., 1990b for details).

Figures 1.8 to 1.10 graph the adjusted means for the three health outcomes, after adjustment for the additive or exposure effects of the risk factors. Comparing Fig. 1.8 to 1.10 to Fig. 1.1 to 1.3, we see that differential levels of exposure to risk factors across age and SES account for a significant portion of the social stratification of aging and health evident in Fig. 1.1 to 1.3. At the younger age levels (25–44), adjusting for differential exposures eliminates all or most of the SES differences in these health outcomes. At the later middle and older age levels (45–75 +) the mean differences between the highest and lowest SES stratum observed in Fig. 1.1 to 1.3 are reduced by about one third (or 25%–40%) in Fig. 1.8 to 1.10. Clearly, differential exposure to these psychosocial risk factors is an important contributor to SES differences in health

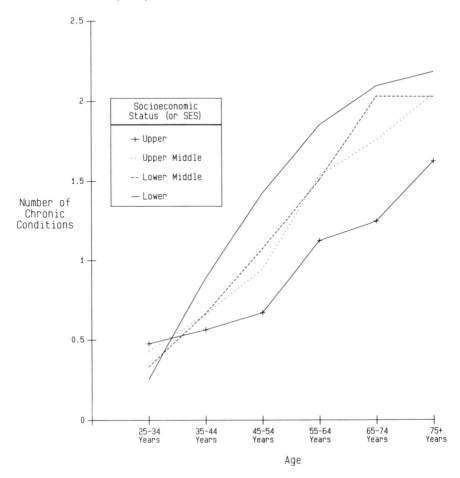

FIG. 1.8.   Age by number of chronic conditions within levels of socioeconomic status controlling for exposure to psychosocial risk factors (see text
for definition of SES levels in terms of education and income). *Source:* House
et al. (1990b). 1986 Americans' Changing Lives Interview Survey data, *n* = 3,617.

beyond age 44, but this exposure cannot explain SES differences fully in this
age range. We have hypothesized that the increasing impact of such risk factors with age (especially perhaps in lower SES groups) may become increasingly important at older age levels.

Differential Impact of Risk Factors by Age as an Explanation.   To test this hypothesis, we have added to the regression equations used to estimate Fig. 1.8–1.10
a set of terms representing the interaction of age and the various risk factors.
Specifically, we have multiplied each risk factor variable by dummy variables

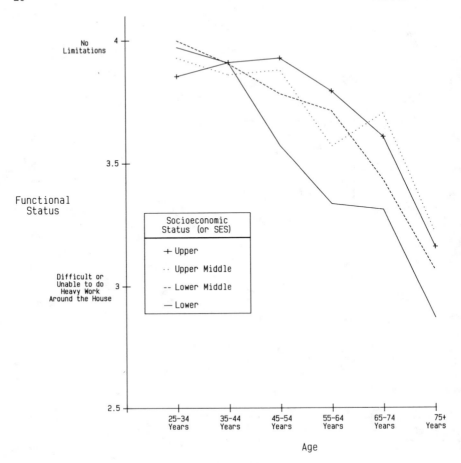

FIG. 1.9. Age by functional status within levels of socioeconomic status, controlling for exposure to psychosocial risk factors (see text for definition of SES levels in terms of education and income). *Source:* House et al. (1990b). 1986 Americans' Changing Lives Interview Survey data, *n* = 3,617.

for the following age groupings: (a) 35–54, (b) 55–74, and (c) 75 +. Adding these product-interaction variables to the additive effects equation tests for variations in the impact (i.e., regression coefficient) of each risk factor across age groups. Five risk factors showed no significant variation in their effects across the age groups (i.e., smoking, marital status, informal and formal social integration, and friend and relative support), but six did (i.e., moderate weight, moderate drinking, chronic financial stress, recent and lifetime life events, and self-efficacy).

Figure 1.11 graphs the variation across age groups in the estimated regression coefficients for the regression of limitation of daily activities on each of

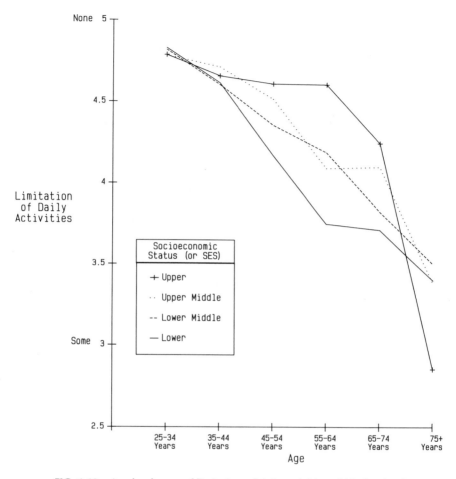

FIG. 1.10. Age by degree of limitation of daily activities within levels of socioeconomic status, controlling for exposure to psychosocial risk factors (see text for definition of SES levels in terms of education and income). *Source:* House et al. (1990b). 1986 Americans' Changing Lives Interview Survey data, *n* = 3,617.

the six risk factors that interacts significantly with age. Although there is not a single invariant pattern to these results, in general the impact of a risk factor variable increases from young adulthood through at least later middle and early old age, with the impact of some continuing to increase into old age, while the impact of others declines in older age (see House et al., 1990b for details on these analyses and similar results for chronic conditions and functional health status). Note that in Fig. 1.11 high values for three risk variables (moderate drinking, self-efficacy, and moderate weight) indicate lower risk. High values for the other three risk variables (number of recent negative life events, num-

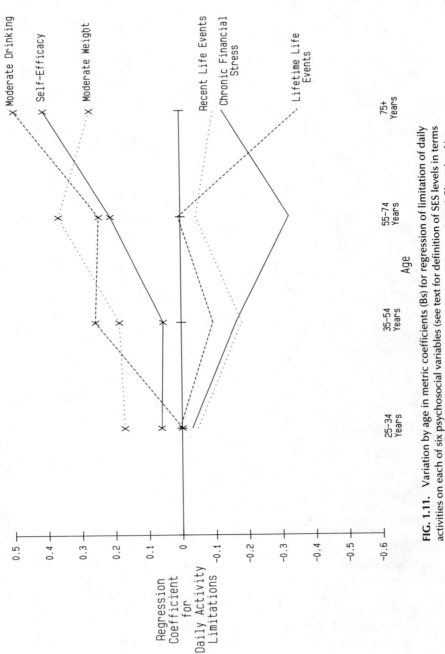

FIG. 1.11. Variation by age in metric coefficients (Bs) for regression of limitation of daily activities on each of six psychosocial variables (see text for definition of SES levels in terms of education and income). *Source:* House et al. (1990b). 1986 Americans' Changing Lives Interview Survey data, $n = 3,617$.

ber of negative lifetime life events, and chronic financial stress) indicate higher risks to health.

This increasing impact of risk factors on health provides a further basis for explaining the social stratification of age and health. SES differences in exposure to risk factors in middle age and early old age have an especially consequential impact on health. Thus, we see the largest SES differentials in health in these age groups because they are characterized by both sizable SES differentials in exposure to risk factors and substantial health impact of the risk factors. In contrast, in early adulthood SES differences in exposure to some risk factors are sizable, but the health impact of the risk factors is muted; and in later old age SES differences in exposure are reduced even if impact remains strong.

Figures 1.12 to 1.14 show the results for limitation of daily activities of adjusting for the interactions representing age differences in the impact of the six risk factors whose impact varied by age, as well as the additive/exposure effects of all 11 risk factors. Comparing these figures to Fig. 1.8 to 1.10 show further reductions in the SES differentials in health, especially in the age range of 55–74. The SES differences in these age groups diminish by a factor of about one third to one half from the differences in Fig. 1.8 to 1.10. Overall, the SES differences across all age groups are reduced by 50%–75% in Fig. 1.12 to 1.14 compared to Fig. 1.1 to 1.3, and the remaining differences are often nonsignificant (see House et al., 1990b for details of these analyses).

We have also tested for SES by risk factor interactions, and three-way interactions among age, SES, and the risk factors. The results are weaker for the SES by risk factor interactions than for the age by risk factor interactions just considered, and even weaker for the three-way interactions. The nature of these effects, however, is as expected: The impact of the risk factors is greater in lower SES groups and among persons who are both older and of lower SES status. We could not estimate all of these interactions in a single equation, but separate analyses of the SES by risk factor and age by SES by risk factor interactions suggest that their inclusion would explain away only a small additional amount of the social stratification of aging and health.

In summary, we find that the combination of differential exposure to risk factors across SES groups and differential impact of the risk factors across age groups substantially explains the social stratification of aging and health. We have omitted from consideration here a number of risk factors which are also likely to play a role—some because they are totally confounded with the dependent variables in cross-sectional analyses (e.g., physical activity), and others because they are not adequately measured in the 1986 ACL survey (e.g., occupational hazards and residues of early life experience). We have explored limited indicators of quantity of medical care, and find little effect of them, which is not surprising because SES differences in access to care have greatly

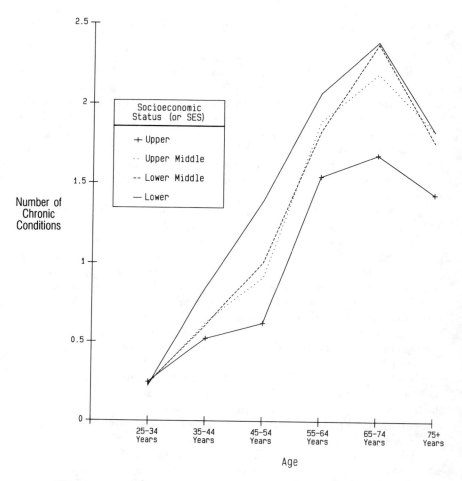

FIG. 1.12. Age by number of chronic conditions within levels of socioeconomic status controlling for exposure to and impact of psychosocial risk factors (see text for definition of SES levels in terms of education and income). *Source:* House et al. (1990b). 1986 Americans' Changing Lives Interview Survey data, *n* = 3,617.

diminished, although not disappeared, since the advent of Medicaid and Medicare (Mechanic, 1968). Differences in the quality or nature of medical care (e.g., preventive vs. therapeutic) remain to be explored. Thus, there is good reason to believe that most, perhaps all, of the social stratification of aging and health is a function of differential exposure to social, psychological, and behavioral risk factors and their differential impact by age (and to a much lesser degree by SES and by the combination of age and SES).

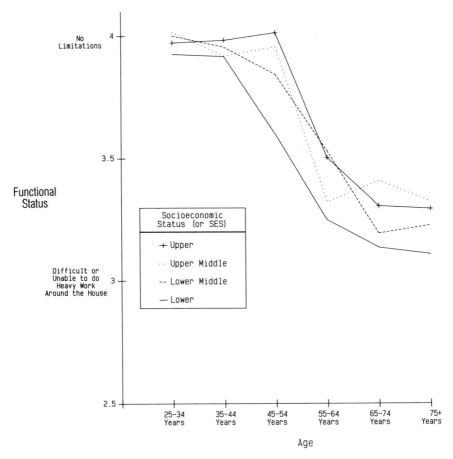

FIG. 1.13. Age by functional status within levels of socioeconomic status, controlling for exposure to and impact of psychosocial risk factors (see text for definition of SES levels in terms of education and income). *Source:* House et al. (1990b). 1986 Americans' Changing Lives Interview Survey data, *n* = 3,617.

DISCUSSION

Some Caveats

As already noted, the largely cross-sectional nature of the data analyzed here makes causal inferences guarded, both in terms of the causal impact of SES (especially income) on health, and in terms of whether the cross-sectional age differences represent a result of aging within individuals or of cohort effects.

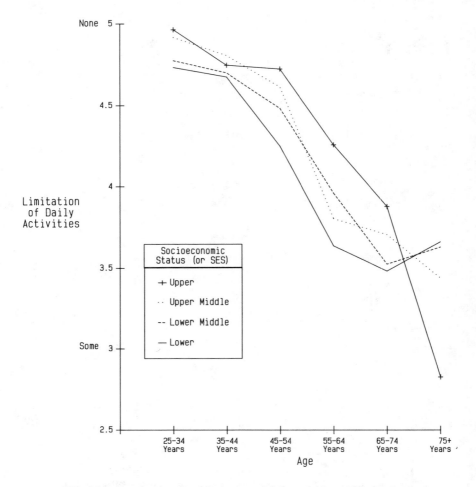

FIG. 1.14. Age by degree of limitation of daily activities within levels of socioeconomic status, controlling for exposure to and impact of psychosocial risk factors (see text for definition of SES levels in terms of education and income). *Source:* House et al. (1990b). 1986 Americans' Changing Lives Interview Survey data, *n* = 3,617.

However, our short-term (2.5 year) longitudinal analyses show both that SES (and education and income considered separately) predict declines in health, especially in later middle age and early old age, and that the psychosocial risk factors considered here also generally predict declines in health. Longer term longitudinal follow-up in the ACL or other data, however, is necessary for firmer causal inference to rule out major cohort effects, and to examine the impact of selective mortality. Similarly, we would like to see extension of the health measures to include direct medical examinations and tests, although such will likely be possible on a representative national sample only in the widely spaced National Health Examination Surveys or in smaller, more intensive local and regional studies.

Nevertheless, we believe the data presented here are most plausibly interpreted as showing that SES is a consequential predictor of how health changes with age, and that this social stratification of aging and health is due primarily to differential exposure to, and impact of, major psychosocial risk factors across SES and age groups. SES differences in health in early middle age primarily reflect SES differences in exposure, differences that tend to diminish in later middle age and old age. However, the impact of these risk factors increases in later middle age and early old age, thus maintaining their contribution to the social stratification of aging and health.

Theoretical and Policy Implications

The results indicate that greater attention to issues of social stratification is essential to understanding and improving health in an increasingly aging society. If lower socioeconomic groups could come to approximate the relationships of age and aging to health that we observe in the upper SES group, we would significantly reduce or postpone many of the health problems of middle age and early old age. Significant health problems will always remain in the last stages of life, but even these may be attenuated in length or intensity if more members of our society approximated the experience of aging and health observed among the most socioeconomically fortunate.

How might this occur? Our theoretical and empirical analyses indicate that variations in exposure to, and the impact of major social, psychological, and behavioral risk factors constitute the mechanisms by which the social stratification of aging and health occurs. Therefore, reducing exposure to, or the impact of, these and related risk factors, especially in middle age and early old age, constitutes a major avenue to modifying the current patterns of social stratification of aging and health. Reducing exposure should be helpful at all ages, while reducing impact (or conversely strengthening resistance or resilience) is more important in later middle age and early old age. These issues are and have been receiving increasing attention in theory, research, and public policy aimed at improving health behaviors, reducing stress, strengthening social relationships and supports, enhancing self-efficacy and improving the immunity, resistance and resilience of human beings in the face of threats to health posed by potentially harmful levels of these or other risk factors (House et al., 1988; Rodin, 1986; Rowe & Kahn, 1987; U.S. Dept. of Health and Human Services, 1988). Our results further support the need for such efforts.

We would close, however, by arguing that social stratification itself must be increasingly central for several reasons in future theory, research, and policy.

First, exposure to almost all major risk factors is stratified by SES, as also is their impact in some cases. Theory, research, and policy on processes of reducing exposure to, or the impact of, major psychosocial risk factors must increasingly be targeted on the lower SES portions of the population where the exposure to and deleterious consequences of these risk factors are greatest. For example, smoking reduction and cessation is increasingly a nonproblematic issue among higher educated and income persons. The variance and potential for change are largely in the lower SES strata.

Such theory, research, and policy must recognize, however, that social stratification is a major causal force producing differential exposure to, and sometimes impact of, these social, psychological, and behavioral risk factors. To a considerable degree people smoke, or fail to eat and drink moderately, or experience stress, lower self-efficacy or poorer social relationships and supports because they are less educated or poor or both. And to say that people are less educated or poor is to say something not only about them as individuals, but more importantly about the social structures and conditions in which they live and work (Kohn & Schooler, 1983). It may be difficult to modify health behaviors, stress, self-attitudes, or social relationships as long as people remain in the same conditions of life and work which foster and maintain these psychosocial risk factors in the first place (Williams, 1990, this volume). The recent examples of cigarette companies targeting Blacks and lower SES females for new brands and special marketing efforts indicate the countervailing forces that confront efforts to reduce smoking in lower SES populations. Further, the risk factors are themselves causally interrelated in complex and not yet fully understood ways. Stress and lack of social relationships and supports and low self-efficacy mutually reinforce each other and may exacerbate problems in health behaviors.

This suggests that theory, research, and policy aimed at eliminating extreme socioeconomic deprivation and moderating socioeconomic inequality may be important and necessary complements to the direct reduction of psychosocial risk factors. Changes in SES can lead to changes in aging and health both through effects on the risk factor mechanisms identified here and through other mechanisms not yet understood or identified. Thus, socioeconomic theory, research, and policy are implicitly or explicitly also exercises in health theory, research, and policy, and can be important adjuncts and complements to them.

Finally, it is important to recognize that even if we were able to explain all of the impact of socioeconomic status on aging and health in terms of intervening psychosocial (or biomedical) risk factors, we cannot disregard socioeconomic status in favor of these mechanisms in doing theory, research, or policy. As Lieberson (1985, chapter 9) has cogently and subtly argued, to identify more proximal intervening variables or mechanisms linking a more distal cause to an outcome is not necessarily to understand the full causal dynamic linking the more distal cause to the outcome. The distal cause may operate to produce the same outcome through different intervening variables or mechanisms at different times or places. If one intervening variable or mechanism is not relevant or operable, another may substitute for it, maintaining equifinality in the link between distal cause and outcome.

The history of the impact of SES on health provides a graphic example of such equifinality in the face of changes in intervening variables and mechanisms. Socioeconomic differentials in morbidity, disability, and mortality have persisted over the past century despite repeated equalization or neutralization of the intervening variables or mechanisms presumably producing that relationship (Antonovsky, 1967). Infectious diseases—once the leading causes of morbidity, disability, and mortality—have been markedly reduced or eradicated, as have SES differentials in sanitation, nutrition, vaccination, and access to medical care; yet the SES differential in health persists virtually undiminished. Chronic diseases and their risk factors have replaced infectious diseases and their risk factors as the major cause of morbidity, disability, and mortality, and have come to be characterized by the same SES gradient.

Over time, socioeconomic differentials in the same disease or risk factor have literally reversed themselves as the disease or risk factor becomes an increasingly important cause of morbidity, disability, and mortality. Earlier in this century smoking, high fat diets, and lack of exercise were more prevalent in high SES groups, but as their impact on health has grown, they have become more prevalent in lower SES groups (cf. Fig. 1.6). Similarly, as various diseases (e.g., coronary heart disease in the first part of the century and AIDS in the last part) have come to be increasingly important sources of morbidity, disability, and mortality, they have gone from initially being more incident and prevalent in higher SES groups to being markedly more incident and prevalent in the lower SES strata (e.g., Marmot et al., 1987; Peterson & Marin, 1988).

In summary, the social stratification of aging and health is arguably a fundamental outcome of our social stratification system itself. Thus, reductions in absolute socioeconomic deprivation or degrees of socioeconomic inequality may in the end be necessary to produce significant and permanent reductions in the social stratification of aging and health. Our data suggest that what is required here is not revolutionary—increasing the percentage of people completing high school and eliminating poverty would significantly reduce if not eliminate these socioeconomic differentials in the relation of aging and health.

In any event, the data presented here suggest that we cannot have cost-effective health research or policy in an increasingly aging society unless we explicitly take account of the social stratification of aging and health. The upper socioeconomic strata in our society appear to be increasingly attaining a life course trajectory of mortality, morbidity, and disability as good as we can humanly hope for, barring a major breakthrough in expanding the finite limits of the human life span. However, we have a major opportunity and responsibility in research and policy to increase the degree to which lower socioeconomic strata experience similar postponement of morbidity and disability into the final years of the human life span.

ACKNOWLEDGMENTS

This chapter was initially prepared for presentation at the Penn State Gerontology Center Conference on Aging, Health Behaviors, and Health Outcomes, Pennsylvania State University, October 23–24, 1989. A revised version was presented at Duke University on March 6, 1990 as part of the Duke University Council on Aging and Human Development Distinguished Faculty Lecture Series. The chapter integrates portions of two other papers (House et al. 1990a and 1990b) and incorporates portions of the text and figures and tables of each. This work has been supported by the National Institute of Aging (Grant # PO1AG05561). We are indebted to Marie Klatt for preparing the manuscript, to Sue Meyer for preparing graphs, to the Technical Sections of the Survey Research Center for the conduct of the sampling, interviewing and coding of the Americans' Changing Lives Survey, and to other colleagues and respondents on the Americans' Changing Lives project for their assistance in various phases of the work. Ronald Abeles and David Featherman provided helpful comments on the initial version of this chapter and numerous other colleagues did likewise on the two papers that are integrated in this chapter.

The 1985 National Health Interview Survey data were made available by the Inter-University Consortium for Political and Social Research (ICPSR). The data for the Health Interview Survey, 1985, were originally collected by the U.S. Department of Health and Human Services and the National Center for Health Statistics. Neither the collector of the original data nor the Consortium bears any responsibility for the analyses or interpretations presented here.

The data computations upon which this chapter is based employed the OSIRIS IV computer software package, which was developed by the Institute for Social Research, The University of Michigan, using funds from the Survey Research Center, Inter-University Consortium for Political Research, National Science Foundation and other sources.

REFERENCES

Antonovsky, A. (1967). Social class, life expectancy, and overall mortality. *Milbank Memorial Fund Quarterly, 45,* 31–73.

Berkman, L. F., & Breslow, L. (1983). *Health and ways of living: The Alameda County Study.* London: Oxford University Press.

Brody, J. A., Brock, D. B., & Williams, T. F. (1987). Trends in the health of the elderly population. *Annual Review of Public Health, 8,* 211–234.

Duncan, G. A., & Smith, K. R. (1989). The rising affluence of the elderly: How far, how fair, and how frail? *Annual Review of Sociology, 15,* 261–289.

Fingerhut, L. A., Wilson, R. W., & Feldheim, J. J. (1980). Health and disease in the United States. *Annual Review of Public Health, 1,* 1–36.

Fox, A. J., Goldblatt, P. O., & Jones, D. R. (1985). Social class mortality differentials: Artifact, selection or life circumstances? *Journal of Epidemiological Community Health, 39,* 1–8.

Fries, J. F. (1980). Aging, natural death, and the compression of morbidity. *New England Journal of Medicine, 303,* 130–135.

Gerontologica Perspecta. (1987). Issue on the compression of morbidity, *1,* 3–66.

Gruenberg, E. (1977). The failure of success. *Milbank Memorial Fund Quarterly, 55,* 3–24.

House, J. S. (1987). Social support and social structure. *Sociological Forum, 2,* 135–146.

House, J. S., Kessler, R. C., Herzog, A. R., Kinney, A. M., Mero, R. P., & Breslow, M. J. (1990a). Age, socioeconomic status, and health. *The Milbank Quarterly, 68,* 383–411.

House, J. S., Kessler, R. C., Herzog, A. R., Kinney, A. M., Mero, R. P., & Breslow, M. J. (1990b). *Socioeconomic status differences in aging and health.* Unpublished manuscript, Institute for Social Research, Ann Arbor, MI.

House, J. S., Kessler, R. C., Herzog, A. R., Kinney, A. M., Mero, R. P., & Breslow, M. J. (1991). *The social stratification of aging and health.* Unpublished manuscript.

House, J. S., Landis, K., & Umberson, D. (1988). Social relationships and health. *Science, 241,* 540–545.

House, J. S., & Robbins, C. (1983). Age, psychosocial stress and health. In M. W. Riley, B. B. Hess, & K. Bond (Eds.), *Aging in society: Selected reviews of recent research.* Hillsdale, NJ: Lawrence Erlbaum Associates.

Kitigawa, E. M., & Hauser, P. M. (1973). *Differential mortality in the United States: A study of socioeconomic epidemiology.* Cambridge, MA: Harvard University Press.

Kohn, M. L., & Schooler, C. (1983). *Work and personality: An inquiry into the impact of social stratification.* Norwood, NJ: Ablex.

Lieberson, S. (1985). *Making it count.* Berkeley: University of California Press.

Manton, K. C. (1982). Changing concepts of morbidity and mortality in the elderly population. *Milbank Memorial Fund Quarterly/Health and Society, 60,* 183–244.

Marmot, M. G., Kogevinas, M., & Elston, M. A. (1987). Social/economic status and disease. *Annual Review of Public Health, 8,* 111–135.

Mechanic, D. (1968). *Medical Sociology.* New York: The Free Press.

National Center for Health Statistics. (1986). *Public use data tape documentation—Parts I, II & III: National Health Interview Survey. 1985.* Hyattsville, MD: National Center for Health Statistics, Public Health Service.

National Center for Health Statistics. (1987). *Health statistics on older persons: United States, 1986—Vital and Health Statistics* (Series 3, No. 25. Public Health Service. DHHS No. (PHS) 87-1409). Washington, DC: U.S. Government Printing Office.

Pearlin, L. I., Lieberman, M. A., Menaghan, E. G., & Mullan, J. T. (1981). The stress process. *Journal of Health and Social Behavior, 22,* 337–356.

Peterson, J. L., & Marin, G. (1988). Issues in the prevention of AIDS among black and hispanic men. *The American Psychologist, 43,* 871–877.

Preston, S. H. (1977). Mortality trends. *Annual Review of Sociology, 3,* 163–178.

Preston, S. H. (1984). Children and the elderly: Divergent paths for America's dependents. *Demography, 21,* 435–458.

Rodin, J. (1986). Aging and health: Effects of the sense of control. *Science, 233,* 1271–1276.

Rodin, J., Schooler, C., & Schaie, K. W. (Eds.). (1990). *Self-directedness: Causes and effects across the life course.* Hillsdale, NJ: Lawrence Erlbaum Associates.

Rosenberg, M. (1965). *Society and the adolescent self-image.* Princeton, NJ: Princeton University Press.

Rowe, J. W., Kahn, R. L. (1987). Human aging: Usual and successful. *Science, 237,* 143–149.

Schneider, E. L., & Brody, J. A. (1983). Aging, natural death and the compression of morbidity: Another view. *New England Journal of Medicine, 309,* 854–857.

Shanas, E., & Maddox, G. L. (1985). Health, health resources, and the utilization of care. In R. H. Binstock & E. Shanas (Eds.), *Handbook of aging and the social sciences* (2nd ed., pp. 697–726). New York: Van Nostrand Reinhold.

Syme, S. L., & Berkman, L. F. (1976). Social class, susceptibility and sickness. *American Journal of Epidemiology, 104,* 1–8.

Theorell, T. G. T. (1982). Review of research on life events and cardiovascular illness. *American Journal of Epidemiology, 104,* 140–147.

Thoits, P. (1983). Dimensions of life events as influences upon the genesis of psychological distress and associated conditions: An evaluation and synthesis of the literature. In H. Kaplan (Ed.), *Psychosocial stress: Trends in theory and research* (pp. 33–103). New York: Academic Press.

U.S. Department of Health and Human Services. (1988). *Promoting health/preventing disease.* Washington, DC: U.S. Department of Health and Human Services.

Verbrugge, L. M. (1984). Longer life but worsening health? Trends in health and mortality of middle-aged and older persons. *Milbank Memorial Fund Quarterly/Health and Society, 62,* 475–519.

Wilkinson, R. G. (1986). Socioeconomic differences in mortality: Interpreting the data on their size and trends. In R. G. Wilkinson (Ed.), *Class and health* (pp. 1–20). London: Tavistock.

Williams, D. R. (1990). Socioeconomic differentials in health: A review and redirection. *Social Psychology Quarterly, 52*(2), 81–99.

Social Stratification and Aging: Contemporaneous and Cumulative Effects

Ronald P. Abeles
National Institute on Aging

In analyzing the interrelationships among social stratification, age, and health, House and his colleagues have taken on an intricate question. What may appear at first glance to be a set of relationships between one societal-level varia- ble (i.e., social stratification) and two person-level variables (i.e., age and health) is at closer inspection even more complicated. The complexity arises from the dual nature of *age* as both a societal- and a person-level variable. On the one hand, age, or better yet, *aging* is a complex biopsychosocial process operating within and upon individuals over their life course. This is the more common way of viewing age. On the other hand, *age* is also a social stratification sys- tem, like class, operating upon socially defined categories of people over histor- ical time. Hence, chronological age is not only a presumed marker of process- es within a person, but also an indication of his/her location within a social system (Riley, Johnson, & Foner, 1972). Thus, House et al. are investigating interactions among two social stratification systems (socioeconomic status and age) and two biopsychosocial processes (health and aging). A formidable task, indeed!

House et al.'s task is made even more difficult by the dynamic nature of these societal- and individual-level processes. It is virtually a truism to note that not only do social systems change over time, but so do individuals. House and his colleagues point to historical changes in societal level processes, which may be "squaring" the morbidity and mortality curves for successive cohorts of Americans and which may be more pronounced among the higher socioeco- nomic strata. Socioeconomic strata differences in health among older people are, according to House et al., the consequences of social stratification processes that differentially (a) place people in opportunity structures (e.g., availability of health care) and (b) inculcate values, attitudes, and behavior patterns (e.g., health- or illness-promoting lifestyles) (Abeles & Riley, 1987).

The dynamic nature of the social stratification and aging processes suggest that they have *contemporaneous* as well as *cumulative* impact on the health of individuals over their life course. That is, a person's location in the age and socioeconomic stratification systems at a particular moment in time affords particular social and economic advantages or disadvantages (e.g., social security benefits). However, as the life-course perspective on aging emphasizes (Abeles & Riley, 1976–1977; Baltes & Goulet, 1970; Baltes & Willis, 1979; Riley, 1979), people have life-long histories of being located in opportunity structures with accumulating impact on their lives, including their health (cf. Abeles, Steel, & Wise, 1980; Hogan, 1978, 1979).

House et al. focus on the contemporaneous impact of socioeconomic status by virtue of classifying people solely in terms of their current income and education. Although educational attainment is relatively constant over the adult life course, income does vary. Thus, in the present cross-sectional analysis, the *life-time* income profile of older people is unknown as is whether their current income in old age represents a significant decrease in economic well-being and socioeconomic status from an earlier period in their lives. Knowledge of income over the life course is important because of the potential influence of income on the person's history of medical care, nutrition, housing quality, and the like, which, in turn, affect life-long patterns of morbidity and ultimately health in old age.

In one way, the cross-sectional analysis of education, as a measure of social stratification, may not misrepresent its cumulative impact over the life course. As a social stratification variable, education takes on significance through the socialization of values, attitudes, and beliefs (Clausen, 1968), which are probably relatively stable over the adult life course (Glenn, 1980; Kinder & Sears, 1985; Sears, 1981). Thus, a current measure of education is probably a reasonable proxy for life-long patterns of attitudes, values, and beliefs, such as sense of personal control (Rodin, 1986a, 1986b), that might influence health-related behaviors and lifestyles and ultimately health per se. As House et al. propose, these attitudinal and behavioral patterns may mediate the effects of a person's socioeconomic status on his or her health.

In another way, however, the cross-sectional analysis of education misses a significant function that education performs in social stratification. Education is a major determinant of an individual's *occupation*, which plays central roles in social stratification and in health. (Indeed, occupation is conspicuously absent *qua* a dimension of social stratification from House et al.'s analyses.) In regard to the former, occupation is a major determinant of social prestige and thereby of how an individual is treated by others (e.g., health-care providers). As for the latter, occupations expose individuals to physical environmental risks to their health (e.g., radiation, chemicals, noise) as well as social environmental risks (e.g., stress). Moreover, the impact of occupations is often cumulative, as has been exemplified in Kohn and Schooler's (1978, 1982) research on the longitudinal impact of occupation on intellectual functioning and personality. Finally, occupation takes on additional significance because of the disjunction in social prestige that accompanies retirement. Retirement brings with it not only a diminution in income, but also the loss of social prestige. It connotes a transition from the valued-role of "worker" to the less-valued or even negatively valued role of "old person" (Butler, 1969, 1989; Riley & Riley, 1989).

Recognizing the distinction between contemporaneous and cumulative effects of socioeconomic status suggests that *change* in status may be a significant contributor to health in old age as a result of stress accompanying *relative deprivation* (Stouffer et al., 1949) and *status incongruity* (Lenski, 1954). As just noted, the transition to old age (i.e., retirement) brings with it a change in income and occupational status. The impact of this change may depend on the person's income and occupational status prior to the transition. For example, both high- and low-income (as determined prior to retirement) older people may experience relatively little alteration in income after retirement in comparison to middle-income individuals. Because earned income represents a smaller percentage of the total income of high socioeconomic status individuals, retirement does not necessarily mean a significant decrease in their standard of living. For lower socioeconomic status individuals, although they are more dependent on earned income, its loss may not markedly change their already low standard of living. (This is not to deny that the loss in earned income may well push many individuals and families over the edge into poverty.) However, middle socioeconomic status people may experience the greatest *relative* loss in standard of living through retirement, because they do not have the cushioning, alternative income sources of higher socioeconomic status people and are not as accustomed to a lower standard of living as are lower socioeconomic status individuals. As a consequence, middle socioeconomic status older people are likely to feel relatively deprived in comparison to their former standard of living and to their still-employed "status equivalents."

As noted earlier, the transition to retirement brings with it changes in income that may affect the opportunity structure aspects of social stratification, such as access to adequate health care, nutrition, and housing. However, because educational attainment is unchanged by the transition to retirement, the socialization aspects of (earlier) socioeconomic status (i.e., values, attitudes, and beliefs) are likely to remain unaltered. This implies that both higher and lower socioeconomic status older people experience little status incongruity between their income and educational statuses. Middle socioeconomic status older people, however, have lost status in terms of income and occupation, while retaining status vis-à-vis education (and the accompanying values, attitudes, and beliefs). Hence, middle socioeconomic status people are likely to experience more stress during the retirement transition because of the resultant status incongruity. This, in turn, suggests possible greater health consequences for middle socioeconomic status older people, at least around the time of retirement, than for other socioeconomic status individuals.

Finally, it should be noted that if the postponement of morbidity is truly more prevalent in higher socioeconomic strata, then a situation is being created where, with each successive birth cohort, there are more and more highly educated people socialized to value productivity, self-efficacy, independence, but who are forced into a role without opportunities for expressing these values (Riley & Riley, 1989). This observation raises questions about the psychological and physical health consequences of such discordance for individuals and about the political consequences for the society as a whole. After all, such relative deprivation and status incongruity is the stuff that revolutions are made of (Abeles, 1976; Runciman, 1968)!

ACKNOWLEDGMENT

While this discussion was written as part of the author's duties as a government employee, the opinions expressed are solely those of the author and do not necessarily reflect the position or policy of the National Institute on Aging.

The advice of Matilda White Riley on an earlier version of these comments is gratefully acknowledged.

REFERENCES

Abeles, R. P. (1976). Relative deprivation, rising expectations, and black militancy. *Journal of Social Issues, 32,* 119–137.

Abeles, R. P., & Riley, M. W. (1976–1977). A life-course perspective on the later years of life: Some implications for research. In *Social Science Research Council Annual Report* (pp. 1–16). New York: Social Science Research Council.

Abeles, R. P., & Riley, M. W. (1987). Longevity, social structure, and cognitive aging. In C. Schooler & K. W. Schaie (Eds.), *Cognitive functioning and social structure over the life course* (pp. 161–175). Norwood, NJ: Ablex.

Abeles, R. P., Steel, L., & Wise, L. L. (1980). Patterns and implications of life-course organization: Studies from Project TALENT. In P. B. Batles & O. G. Brim Jr. (Eds.), *Life-span development and behavior* (pp. 308–337). New York: Academic Press.

Baltes, P. B., & Goulet, L. R. (1970). Status and issues of a life-span developmental psychology. In L. R. Goulet & P. B. Baltes (Eds.), *Life-span developmental psychology* (pp. 4–23). New York: Academic Press.

Baltes, P. B., & Willis, S. L. (1979). Life-span developmental psychology, cognitive functioning, and social policy. In M. W. Riley (Ed.), *Aging from birth to death: Interdisciplinary perspectives* (pp. 15–46). Boulder, CO: Westview Press.

Butler, R. N. (1969). Ageism: Another form of bigotry. *Gerontologist, 9,* 243–246.

Butler, R. N. (1989). Dispelling ageism: The cross-cutting intervention. *The Annals of the American Academy of Political and Social Science, 503,* 138–147.

Clausen, J. A. (Ed.). (1968). *Socialization and society.* Boston: Little, Brown.

Glenn, N. D. (1980). Values, attitudes, and beliefs. In O. G. Brim Jr. & J. Kagan (Eds.), *Constancy and change in human development* (pp. 596–640). Cambridge, MA: Harvard University Press.

Hogan, D. (1978). Order of events in the life course. *American Sociological Review, 48,* 573–586.

Hogan, D. (1979). *The transition to adulthood as a career contingency.* Paper presented at the Rural Sociological Society, Burlington, VT.

Kinder, D. R., & Sears, D. O. (1985). Public opinion and political action. In G. Lindzey & E. Aronson (Eds.), *The handbook of social psychology* (pp. 659–742). New York: Random House.

Kohn, M. L., & Schooler, C. (1978). The reciprocal effects of the substantive complexity of work and intellectual flexibility: A longitudinal assessment. *American Journal of Sociology, 84,* 24–52.

Kohn, M. L., & Schooler, C. (1982). Job conditions and personality: A longitudinal assessment of their reciprocal effects. *American Journal of Sociology, 87,* 1257–1286.

Lenski, G. (1954). Status crystallization: A nonvertical dimension of social status. *American Sociological Review, 19,* 405–413.

Riley, M. W. (1979). Introduction: Life-course perspectives. In M. W. Riley (Ed.), *Aging from birth to death: Interdisciplinary perspectives* (pp. 3–14). Boulder, CO: Westview Press.

Riley, M. W., Johnson, M. J., & Foner, A. (1972). *Aging and society.* New York: Russell Sage.

Riley, M. W., & Riley, J. W., Jr. (1989). The lives of older people and changing social roles. *The Annals of the American Academy of Political and Social Science, 503,* 14–28.

Rodin, J. (1986a). Aging and health: Effects of the sense of control. *Science, 233,* 1271–1276.

Rodin, J. (1986b). Health, control, and aging. In M. M. Baltes & P. B. Baltes (Eds.), *The psychology of control and aging* (pp. 139–165). Hillsdale, NJ: Lawrence Erlbaum Associates.

Runciman, W. G. (1968). *Relative deprivation and social justice.* London: Routledge & Kegan Paul.

Sears, D. O. (1981). Life-stage effects on attitude change, especially among the elderly. In S. B. Kiesler, J. N. Morgan, & V. K. Oppenheimer (Eds.), *Social change* (pp. 183–204). New York: Academic Press.

Stouffer, S. A., Lumsdaine, M., Williams, R., Smith, M. B., Janis, I., Star, S., & Cottrell, L. (1949). *The American soldier.* New Brunswick, NJ: Princeton University Press.

2

Socioeconomic Status, Health Behaviors, and Health Status Among Blacks

Sherman A. James
Nora L. Keenan
Steve Browning
University of North Carolina

INTRODUCTION

Black Americans are a large, diverse, and still rapidly growing racial minority group. In separate analyses of the changing demographics of U.S. Blacks since the early 1970s, O'Hare (1987) and Jackson (1988) called attention not only to the rapid growth of the Black population but also to the rapid aging of the U.S. Black population. Concerning population size increases, the U.S. Census Bureau in 1986 estimated the Black population at 29.4 million persons, or 12.2% of the total U.S. population. This compared to the 26.8 million, or 11.8%, who were counted in 1980, and the 22.5 million, or 11.1%, who were counted in 1970 (O'Hare, 1987).

The aging of the Black population is indicated by the steady rise in the median age of Blacks: 22.4 years in 1970; 24.9 years in 1980; and 26.3 years in 1984 (O'Hare, 1987). The proportion of the Black population classified as elderly (i.e., age 65 plus) grew by 31.9% during the 1970s; and between 1980–1986 the number of Blacks age 85 and over grew by an impressive 33.9% (O'Hare, 1987). The Census Bureau projects a continued increase in the number of Black and White elderly through the year 2020. By the year 2000, the White elderly is expected to increase by 22.7% and the Black elderly is expected to increase by 45.6% (Jackson, 1988).

Projections concerning the health status of the Black population relative to the White during this period cannot be made with the same confidence. There are already some indications, however, that the current racial disparities in health will remain constant, if they do not actually increase, in the years ahead. The factors responsible for this gloomy prediction include the greater ease with which the White population, especially those of middle-class standing, can adopt healthier lifestyles while young, and maintain such lifestyles throughout early and middle adulthood, thereby possibly postponing the onset of degenerative diseases like hypertension, heart disease, and diabetes until late adulthood (Guralnik & Kaplan, 1989; Sempos, Cooper, Kovar, & McMiller, 1988; Wing, 1988).

It seems self-evident that the socioeconomic position of Blacks relative to that of Whites will be a major determinant of how large the health differential between the races will be in the years ahead. It is likely that the geographical location of blacks (i.e., whether they live in the Northeast or on the West Coast, in central cities or the suburbs) will also influence this health differential (Wing, 1988). With this in mind, we would like to offer a research example from the Southeastern region of the United States, specifically eastern North Carolina, which might illustrate some of the challenges researchers may face in studying aging and health in Blacks. Although this research example comes from a fairly typical, nonmetropolitan biracial community in the South, we do not claim that the findings apply to communities other than the one studied.

METHODS

Study Setting

The study setting is Edgecombe County, North Carolina, a poor, predominantly rural community in the northeast section of the state. In 1980, the Department of Epidemiology at The University of North Carolina in Chapel Hill, received an NIH grant[1] to develop, implement, and evaluate a series of pilot programs to control high blood pressure in this community. Edgecombe County is part of the so-called "stroke death belt," a section of the Coastal Plains region of the Carolinas and Georgia that for decades has reported higher cerebrovascular death rates than any other part of the country (Heyman et al., 1976). The county's adult population in 1980 was 46% Black, according to the U.S. Census; and developing programs to reach Black hypertensives (especially Black male hypertensives) was a major objective of this hypertension control program (James et al., 1984; Wagner et al., 1984).

Sampling and Data Collection

Edgecombe County is comprised of 14 townships, each containing varying numbers of persons and households. To ensure adequate representation of all geographic areas, a stratified (by township) random sample of 1,000 households

[1]NHLBI Grant No. HL 24003.

TABLE 2.1
The Study Sample: Edgecombe County, NC 1980

	N	%
White men	507	25.0
White women	578	28.5
Black men	372	18.3
Black women	573	28.2
Total	2030	100%

was obtained, with proportional representation of households across townships (Wagner et al., 1984). Local interviewers were hired and trained in survey methods; questionnaire administration; and in the measurement of height, weight, and blood pressure. The interview lasted about 1 hour, and was conducted in the respondent's home by an interviewer of the same race for approximately 85% of households. Interviews were sought from all persons 18 years of age and older in the household.

The field work began in January 1980 and was concluded in September 1980. There were 2,030 individuals interviewed, with an overall response of 91%. Response levels varied from a high of 95% for White women to a low of 82% for Black men. The response for Black women was 92%; for White men 88%.

The Study Sample: Race, Age, and SES Characteristics

Table 2.1 summarizes the race–gender composition of the 2,030 respondents. As in the county as a whole, Blacks comprised 46% of the study participants. The number of Black men, however, is relatively small—only 372. When stratified by other variables of interest, this small number will impose some constraints on data analysis options. Analytic constraints of a more general nature also exist because this sample was not specifically drawn to investigate age, race, and SES influences on health and health behaviors. Two major constraints are: (a) small numbers of persons over age 65 for all four race–gender groups,[2] and (b) severely restricted variation on socioeconomic status (SES) indicators such as education, occupation, and income for Blacks, especially Blacks over 50 years of age.

The first constraint—few persons over age 65—led to the decision to create just three age groups, with the first group consisting of persons age 55 and older, a second group consisting of persons 35-54 years of age, and a third group consisting of persons 18-34 years of age. The distribution of the four

---

[2]Among persons age 65 plus, there were 100 White women, 80 Black women, 58 White men, and 59 Black men.

race–gender groups across these three age categories is summarized in Table 2.2. Although not ideal, these age categories seemed a reasonable way to distinguish young adulthood, herein defined by ages 18–34, and the middle and later stages of adulthood, herein defined by the age categories 35–54 and 55 plus, respectively. The small number of individuals over age 65 precludes separate analysis of the elderly within the category of later adulthood. As can be seen in Table 2.2, the percent distribution of individuals across the three age categories is fairly comparable for Whites. Although these percentages are not unduly disproportionate for Blacks, there are proportionately more 18- to 34-year-old Blacks in the sample than Blacks 35 and older.

The second major constraint—restricted variation on SES for Blacks as compared to Whites—also had important analytic implications. Race–gender-specific distributions for education, occupation, and total family income revealed the expected Black disadvantages across all three age categories. However, racial inequalities on these SES indicators were sufficiently great for the two older age categories that age-specific racial comparisons on health outcomes and health behaviors that are known to be strongly associated with SES were considered methodologically inappropriate.

Comparing age-related differences in health and health behaviors between men and women of the same race was one alternative strategy considered because it circumvents the problem of residual confounding by SES. This, too, proved unattractive, however, because age-related gender differences in family and work roles complicate the interpretation of observed gender differences in health behaviors such as cigarette smoking and alcohol consumption, just

TABLE 2.2
The Edgecombe County Study Sample, 1980:
Age–Race–Gender Composition

Age	White Males		Black Males	
	N	%	N	%
18–34	177	35	172	46
35–54	177	35	97	26
55 plus	153	30	103	28
Totals	507	100	372	100

Age	White Females		Black Females	
	N	%	N	%
18–34	190	33	240	42
35–54	197	34	170	30
55 plus	191	33	163	28
Totals	578	100	573	100

TABLE 2.3
The Edgecombe County Study Sample, 1980:
Education by Age–Race–Gender

	White Males		Black Males	
	<HS	≥HS	<HS	≥HS
Age	N	N	N	N
18–34	46	131	66	106
35–54	80	97	82	15
55 plus	97	56	97	6
Totals	223	284	245	127

	White Females		Black Females	
	<HS	≥HS	<HS	≥HS
Age	N	N	N	N
18–34	44	146	79	161
35–54	73	124	118	52
55 plus	102	89	163	24
Totals	219	359	336	237

as age-related biological differences between men and women complicate the interpretation of gender differences in risk for health problems like hypertension and obesity. These substantive concerns, along with a perceived need for more basic, descriptive work in this area, argued for using race and gender-specific analytic models. In such models, Black women are compared only to other Black women, White men only to other White men, and so forth. Thus, although the opportunity to make formal statistical comparisons *across* race and gender groups is lost with this modeling strategy, such loss is partially compensated for by the improved interpretability of effect modification, by SES, of any observed age differences in health and health behaviors for a given race–gender group. Of course, general patterns in the data that transcend race or gender may still be discernible.

Education was chosen as the SES indicator for this study. Race–gender differences in educational achievement, at least up to high school, were less marked than for either occupation or total family income. Moreover, total family income was not adjusted for family size, and occupation had more missing values, especially for women. Beyond these considerations, education has been widely used as an indicator of SES in epidemiologic studies of coronary heart disease risk factors such as hypertension, obesity, smoking, and exercise (Liberatos, Link, & Kelsey, 1988).

Table 2.3 summarizes the educational characteristics (high school vs. non-high school) of the study sample stratified by age, race, and gender. Education and age are highly correlated with each other, especially for Blacks. The small number of high school graduates among older Black men will obviously preclude the reliable estimation of age by education interactions within this race–gender group.

Health Behaviors

The health behaviors studied are cigarette smoking and recreational physical exercise. If respondents answered "yes" to the question "Do you now smoke cigarettes?" they were classified as smokers. If they said they do not exercise for fun or fitness, they were classified as "non-exercisers." The study of alcohol consumption, another major health behavior, was also of interest. However, the low prevalence of daily drinkers for all race, gender, and age groups in the sample plus the lack of information on type and quantities of alcohol typically consumed, did not permit an unambiguously high-risk group for alcohol-related health problems to be identified. Hence, it was decided to treat alcohol consumption as a covariate only when examining health outcomes such as hypertension. To facilitate this, response options for the alcohol question were dichotomized into "frequent drinkers" and "others," with the former designating persons who drink alcoholic beverages at least once a week. Defined in this manner, "frequent drinking" cannot be presumed to represent a problematic health behavior.

Health Outcomes

The health outcomes of interest are hypertension, obesity, and Poor/Fair Self-Rated Health. Three sitting blood pressures were taken on each individual. If the average of the second and third diastolic pressures was greater than or equal to 90 mmHg, or the individual was currently taking anti-hypertensive drugs, he or she was classified as hypertensive. Obesity was defined as a body mass index (BMI) greater than 31.4 for females or 31.8 for males. These BMI cutpoints approximate the 95th percentiles in NHANES I (Cohen et al., 1987) and also indicate 140%, or more, ideal body weights using 1983 Metropolitan Life Insurance Height/Weight tables. These cutpoints, therefore, denote fairly serious levels of obesity. Self-rated health was measured by the Rand Corporation's nine-item Current Health Scale (Ware & Davies-Avery, 1978). Two sample items from this scale are: "According to the doctors I've seen, my health is now excellent"; and "I feel about as good now as I ever have." The five response options per question were: "false," "mostly false," "don't know," "mostly true," and "true." Responses indicating good health received higher scores, with total scores ranging from a low of 9 to a high of 45. A score less than 24 indicates that, on average, the individual said "mostly false" or "don't know" to statements suggesting good health status, or "mostly true" or "don't know" to statements suggesting poor health status. Such individuals were classified as having "poor/fair" self-rated health.

Data Analyses

For each race–gender group, logistic regression (Kleinbaum, Kupper, & Morgenstern, 1982) was used to estimate associations between age, education, and the indicated health outcomes and behaviors. Parameters for the logistic models were estimated by a method of maximum likelihood (Harrel, 1980). For cigarette smoking and physical exercise, the models included terms for age, education, and an age by education product term. Age was defined by two dummy variables; the first contrasted 35- to 54-year-olds to 18- to 34-year-olds, and the second contrasted persons 55 and older to those 18–34. Education was also defined by a dummy variable, high school graduate versus nongraduate. If no significant age by education interactions were observed, this product term was dropped from the model (Kleinbaum et al., 1982). If interaction (i.e., $p < .05$) was observed, however, its magnitude and direction were studied by choosing 18- to 34-year-old non-high school graduates as the referent group and, through a series of five dummy variables, contrasting scores on the relevant health behavior for this group to that of the other five age-education subgroups.

The models for obesity and poor/fair self-rated health included the same three previously mentioned terms. Obesity was studied only in women because, in this sample, it was relatively uncommon among men. Models estimating the prevalence of hypertension likewise included variables for age, education, and an age by education product term. However, in predicting hypertension status, terms for obesity (coded 1 vs. 0), alcohol consumption (frequent = 1, other = 0), and physical exercise (non-exerciser = 1, exerciser = 0), all established risk factors for hypertension, were included in the models. In the interest of parsimony, the results for Black men and White men are presented in the same graphs, as are the results for Black women and White women. But, again, only within race–gender comparisons are appropriate.

RESULTS

Figure 2.1 presents race-specific prevalences of cigarette smoking among males; the data are further stratified by age and education. Data for Whites are represented by open circles and squares, and for Blacks by closed circles and

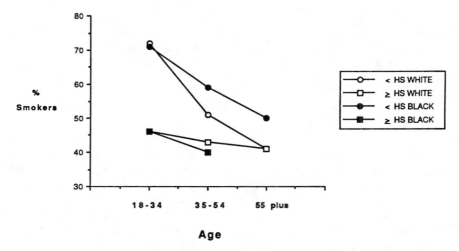

FIG. 2.1. Percent smokers by age, race, and education : Males (Edgecombe County, North Carolina, 1980).

squares. For both racial groups, non-high school graduates are represented by circles, and high school graduates by squares. Because there were only six Black men ages 55 plus who had graduated from high school, their data are not shown on this nor subsequent graphs. For Black men, a strong education effect (β = 1.1, s.e. = .33, p < .002) was observed for cigarette smoking, with non-high school graduates being more likely to smoke cigarettes (at every age) than high school graduates. The prevalence of cigarette smoking among young, less well-educated Black men was 71%. For White men, a strong age by education interaction on smoking was observed, with the 72% prevalence of cigarette smoking shown here for the 18- to 34-year-old non-high school graduates being significantly higher (p < .01) than the prevalence of cigarette smoking in all other groups of White men.

Figure 2.2 presents smoking data for women. As for White men, a strong age by education interaction was observed for White women. The 64% prevalence of cigarette smoking among 18- to 34-year-old non-high school graduates was significantly higher (p < .001) than the prevalence observed for all other subgroups of White women. Neither age nor education significantly influenced cigarette smoking among Black women.

Figure 2.3 presents data on physical exercise for men. Among White men, the percent of non-exercisers increased significantly with age (e.g., β = −1.2, s.e. = .33, p < .001 for 18- to 34-year-olds vs. 35- to 54-year-olds). Also, non-high school graduates were significantly (β = −.95, s.e. = .41, p < .02) less likely to engage in physical exercise than were high school graduates. For Black men, the seemingly large educational differences in physical exercise

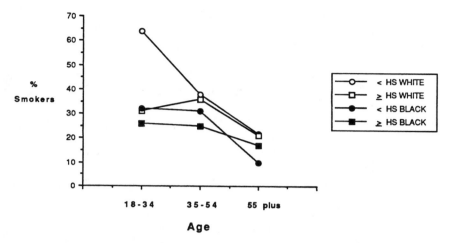

FIG. 2.2. Percent smokers by age, race, and education : Females (Edgecombe County, North Carolina, 1980).

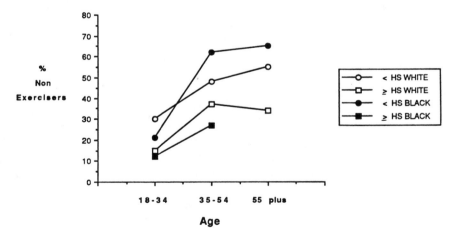

* **Persons who do not exercise for fun or fitness.**

FIG. 2.3. Percent non-exercisers* by age, race, and education : Males (Edgecombe County, North Carolina, 1980).

(especially for the 35- to 54-year-old men) were not statistically significant, primarily because of the small number of better educated Black men in the older age groups.

As was observed for White men, age and education were independently associated with physical exercise among White women (Fig. 2.4). The percent of non-exercisers increased significantly with age (e.g., $\beta = -1.1$, s.e. $= .29$, $p < .001$ for 18- to 34-year-olds vs. ages 35–54). Also non-high school graduates were somewhat less likely ($\beta = -.71$, s.e. $= .40$, $p < .07$) to engage in physical exercise than high school graduates. For Black women, a significant education effect ($\beta = .59$, s.e. $= .29$, $p < .04$) on physical exercise was observed, with non-exercise levels reaching 71% in the oldest group of non-high school graduates. A significant age effect ($\beta = -.82$, s.e. $= .33$, $p < .01$) on physical exercise was also observed among Black women, but this was limited to the contrast between 35- to 54-year-olds and 18- to 34-year-olds. Indeed, relative to other subgroups of Black women, high school graduates ages 55 plus reported fairly low levels of non-exercise.

Obesity (Fig. 2.5) was the first of three health outcomes to be examined. Among White women, the prevalence of obesity did not vary significantly by age or education. Indeed, there was remarkably little variation in obesity, by age, for high school graduates. For Black women, however, age was strongly associated with obesity, especially for the contrast involving 18- to 34-year-olds versus women 55 plus ($\beta = 1.38$, s.e. $= .46$, $p < .003$). For the 35- to 54-year-old non-high school graduates, the prevalence of obesity was nearly 50%. Finally, although not statistically significant, the educational "cross-over"

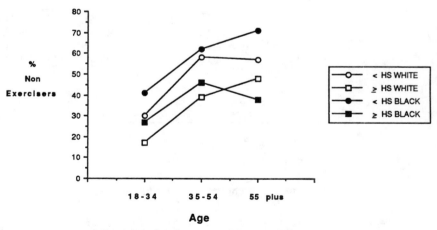

* Persons who do not exercise for fun or fitness.

FIG. 2.4. Percent non-exercisers* by age, race, and education : Females (Edgecombe County, North Carolina, 1980).

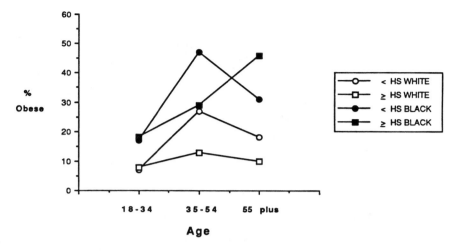

FIG. 2.5. Percent obese* by age, race, and education: Females (Edgecombe County, North Carolina, 1980)

in the prevalence of obesity among Black women age 55 plus suggests that the relatively low levels of physical inactivity shown for high school graduates in the previous figure may be related to their recognition of being seriously overweight.

The adjusted prevalences of hypertension for men are shown in Fig. 2.6. Strong age effects (e.g., β = 1.23, s.e. = .35, p < .0004 for 18- to 34-year-olds vs. persons 55 plus) were observed for Black men, with hypertension prevalences increasing sharply with the onset of middle age. The differences by education, although consistent across age groups, were not statistically significant. These age effects, it should be noted, were independent of body mass index, alcohol consumption and physical exercise. For White men, strong age effects (e.g., β = 1.24, s.e. = .33, p < .0002 for 18- to 34-year-olds vs. persons 35–54) were also observed. Lack of physical exercise was also significantly associated (β = − .53, s.e. = .23, p < .02) with hypertension in White men, but the age effects—by far the strongest predictor in the model—were independent of physical activity, body mass index and alcohol consumption. Education was clearly unrelated to hypertension prevalence in White men.

For Black women, the increase in hypertension prevalence (Fig. 2.7) with age (e.g., β = 1.97, s.e. = .33, p < .00001 for 18- to 34-year-olds vs. 35- to 54-year-olds) was striking. Nearly two thirds of all Black women ages 55 plus were hypertensive. This significant age effect was independent of body mass index, alcohol consumption, and physical exercise. These same conclusions

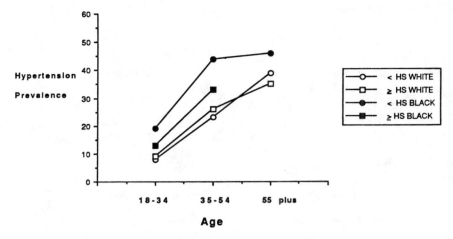

* Diastolic Blood Pressure ≥ 90 mmHg, or treated.

** Adjusted within race-specific logistic regression models that included terms for age, education, BMI, alcohol consumption, and physical exercise.

FIG. 2.6.   Hypertension* prevalence** by age, race, and education : Males (Edgecombe County, North Carolina, 1980).

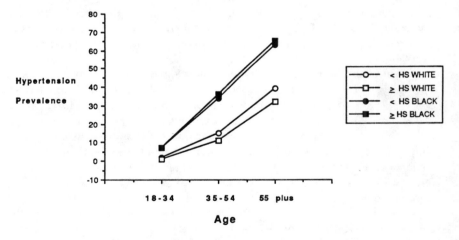

* Diastolic Blood Pressure ≥ 90 mmHg, or treated.

** Adjusted within race-specific logistic regression models that included terms for age, education, BMI, alcohol consumption, and physical exercise.

FIG. 2.7.   Hypertension* prevalence** by age, race, and education: Females (Edgecombe County, North Carolina, 1980).

hold for White women. Hypertension prevalence rose steadily with age and this significant age effect (e.g., β = 2.5, s.e. = .75, p < .001 for 18- to 34-year-olds vs. persons 35–54) was independent of body mass index, alcohol consumption, and physical exercise.

Figure 2.8 presents the findings on poor/fair self-rated health for men. Strong age effects (e.g., β = 1.17, s.e. = .51, p < .02 for 18- to 34-year-olds vs. persons 35–54) were observed for White men; however the apparent differences by education were not statistically significant. No statistically significant age or education effects were observed for Black men. One can speculate, however, that the linear increase in poor/fair self-rated health with age for non-high school graduates—in contrast to the apparent absence of a similar increase for high school graduates—would have produced a strong age by education interaction had this sample contained a larger number of older, better educated Black men.

Figure 2.9 presents comparable data on self-rated health for women. For White women, the percent scoring in the "poor/fair" range increased in linear fashion with age (e.g., β = 1.1, s.e. = .40, p < .01 for 18- to 34-year-olds vs. persons 35–54). Differences by education, however, were not statistically significant. Among Black women, significant age (e.g., β = .74, s.e. = .38, p < .05 for 18- to 34-year-olds vs. persons 35–54) and education (β = .73, s.e. = .34, p < .03) main effects were observed, with a high school education as

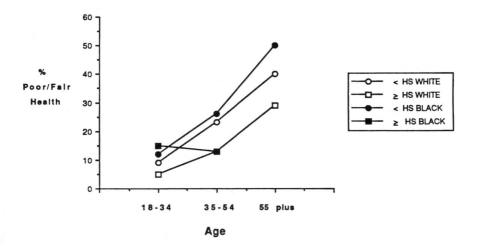

* Score < 24 on the Rand Corporation's Current Health Scale
(Maximum score = 45)

FIG. 2.8. Percent pool/fair self-rated* health by age, race, and education: Males (Edgecombe County, North Carolina, 1980).

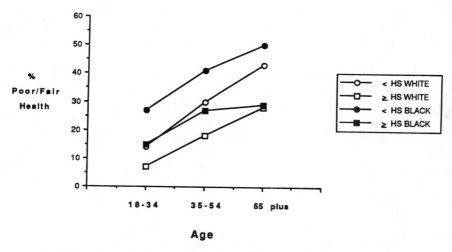

* Score < 24 on the Rand Corporation's Current Health Scale
(Maximum score = 45)

FIG. 2.9. Percent poor/fair self-rated* health by age, race, and education: Females (Edgecombe County, North Carolina, 1980).

well as youthful age being associated with lower prevalences of poor/fair self-rated health.

Table 2.4 provides a summary of the major study findings for the two health behaviors, cigarette smoking and physical exercise. For Whites, the pattern of associations is the same for men and women. For example, although 18- to 34-year-olds were much more likely to smoke cigarettes than the two older age groups, this ''excess prevalence'' of cigarette smoking in the young was largely concentrated among non-high school graduates. And, although persons over age 35 were less likely to engage in recreational exercise than younger adults, non-high school graduates were less likely to be exercisers at all ages. For Blacks, the pattern of significant associations differs for men and women. Among women, those between 35–54 years of age were less likely than their younger counterparts to engage in recreational exercise, and non-high school graduates at all ages were less likely to do so. Smoking was unrelated to age and education among Black women. For Black men, cigarette smoking was strongly associated with educational achievement. Differences by education in physical exercise were also noted for Black men but these differences did not reach statistical significance.

A summary of the significant findings for the three health outcomes is presented in Table 2.5. The pattern of results is quite clear. For Whites, age is a strong correlate of both hypertension and poor/fair self-rated health. No significant differences by level of education were observed. Neither age nor

TABLE 2.4
Subgroups at Highest Risk on Selected Health Behaviors

Race to Gender	Cigarette Smokers	Non-Exercisers
White men		
	non-HS graduates under age 35	non-HS graduates and persons over age 35
White women		
	non-HS graduates under age 35	non-HS graduates and persons over age 35
Black men	non-HS graduates	
Black women		non-HS graduates and persons ages 35–54

education was associated with obesity in White women. Age was strongly associated with obesity in Black women, and was also a strong predictor of hypertension status and poor/fair self-rated health in this group. Among Black women, non-high school graduates were also more likely to be classified as being in poor/fair health. As for Whites and Black women, age was an important correlate of hypertension status in Black men.

TABLE 2.5
Subgroups at Highest Risk on Selected Health Outcomes

Race–Gender	Obesity	Hypertension	Fair/Poor Self-Rated Health
White men	NA		
		persons over age 35	persons over age 35
White women			
		persons over age 35	persons over age 35
Black men	NA		
		persons over age 35	
Black women			
	persons over age 35	persons over age 35	persons over age 35 and non-HS graduates

DISCUSSION

Despite the limitations in study design, these findings have several important implications. First, socioeconomic status, herein measured by level of education, is clearly relevant to understanding within group variation in important health behaviors like cigarette smoking and physical exercise in this biracial, southern community. Indeed, the very high prevalences of cigarette smoking among younger, less well-educated Whites and among all less well-educated Black men—a full 16 years after the Surgeon General's initial warning against cigarette smoking—is a cause for concern. In the years since 1980, anti-smoking educational campaigns and broad-scaled environmental interventions such as the initiation of no-smoking areas in public settings may help reduce cigarette smoking in this young cohort over time. Even so, the long-term risks to their health, attributable to cigarette smoking while young, may not be trivial.

Differences in physical exercise by age and education were also apparent and such differences point to the potential influence of social structure on the likelihood of maintaining a healthy lifestyle. For example, the observed educational differences in physical exercise for Whites, and for Black women, were probably influenced, at least in part, by differential placement in the occupational structure. Individuals in this community with less than a high school education were much more likely to be employed in manual, physically taxing jobs. The resulting physical fatigue and musculoskeletal discomforts are likely to be a disincentive for them to engage in physical exercise during their leisure time. Education was less strongly associated with skilled level employment for Black men. This, plus the problem of small numbers, probably explains the nonsignificant effect of education on physical exercise observed for Black men.

The increasing prevalence of physical inactivity with age across race–gender–age groups is also a matter of concern. Although it is true that the increasing prevalence of chronic disease and functional disabilities with age render physical exercise less manageable for many older people, one cannot but wonder if physical inactivity among older adults, especially in low SES communities, is not made worse by the absence in the mass media of effective role models over 50 years of age. While the entire American population is becoming more health conscious about regular exercise for weight control and cardiovascular fitness, there are still many groups within the society who remain unexposed to health promotion messages about affordable recreational exercise that one can engage in after 40–50 years of age.

Successful weight control throughout the life cycle is difficult for most people; and national data (NIH, 1985), as well as data from this study, indicate that this is especially difficult for adult Black women. As Kumanyika (1987) pointed out, excess obesity in Black females is not observed until adolescence. Moreover, low SES is a strong risk indicator for the onset of obesity in Black women. Data from this study confirm the strong association between obesity and age in Black women but our data provide no additional insights into factors that might be responsible for this association. Detailed studies of environmental, behavioral, and biological risk factors for obesity in Black women are clearly needed since successful weight control could impact significantly on the life expectancy of middle-aged Black women (Guralnik & Kaplan, 1989; Lubben, Weiler, & Chi, 1989).

Age was a strong predictor of hypertension prevalence in all four race–gender groups in this study, with adjusted hypertension prevalences among Black women, ages 55 plus, approaching 65%. The age effects observed in this study, as in most studies, could not be accounted for by education, physical exercise, or alcohol consumption. It should be noted, however, that increases in blood pressure after early adulthood are not an inevitable biological consequence of aging (Cassel, 1975; James, 1987). Rather, such increases probably result from a complex interplay among dietary factors, lack of weight control, and chronic exposure to difficult social and economic stressors (Strogatz & James, 1986; James, Strogatz, Wing, & Ramsey, 1987), the net impact of which may be permanent structural changes in the homeostatic mechanisms that regulate blood pressure (Obrist, 1981). None of these important dimensions of SES was explored in the current study, but several of them are now under investigation by our group in an ongoing study of social, behavioral, and environmental risk factors in Black hypertension.[3]

Finally, age was a significant predictor of poor/fair self-rated health in all groups except Black men. For Black women, lack of a high school education was also a strong predictor of perceived poorer health status. This subjective measure of health was included in order to assess health status in a more global manner than specific indicators like hypertension and obesity would permit. Individual responses to items in the Current Health Scale may have been influenced by unconscious processes (e.g., social desirability) as well as by conscious awareness of chronic health problems, financial worries, and impaired social relationships (Anderson, Mullner, & Cornelius, 1987). Nevertheless, this kind of global health measure may be a useful indicator of overall ''quality of life'' or, in the context of research on aging, a useful indicator of ''successful'' aging (Rowe & Kahn, 1987). The fact that self-perceptions of being in poor/fair health increased so sharply with age in this population, and did so by early middle age for most groups, suggests that postponing age-related decrements in subjective well-being will not be easy in this and similarly economically disadvantaged populations.

The cross-sectional design of this study imposes certain obvious limitations. Longitudinal studies that eliminate or minimize these limitations (including small numbers of Blacks over age 60) are clearly needed. One such longitudinal study is now underway (House et al., chapter 1, this volume). The formu-

---

[3]The Pitt County Hypertension Project, NIH Grant No. HL 33211.

lation of sound national policy to improve the health of the elderly, including the Black elderly, must be based on comprehensive studies of high quality. This conference will be an important step toward achieving this goal.

ACKNOWLEDGMENTS

The authors thank David Strogatz and Joann Garrett-Mills for their constructive critique of this chapter, and Julie Gazmararian and Joann Crescio for their assistance in preparing the manuscript.

REFERENCES

Andersen, R. M., Mullner, R. M., & Cornelius, L. J. (1987). Black–white differences in health status: Methods or substance? *The Milbank Quarterly, 65*(1), 72–99.

Cassell, J. C. (1975). Studies of hypertension in migrants. In O. Paul (Ed.), *Epidemiology and control of hypertension* (pp. 41–61). New York: Stratton Intercontinental Medical Book Corporation.

Cohen, B. B., Barbano, H. E., Cox, C. S., Feldman, J. J., Finucane, F. F., Kleinman, J. C., & Madans, J. H. (1987). *Plan and operation of the NHANES I Epidemiologic Follow-up Study, 1982–84* (DHHS Publication No. (PHS) 87-1324). Washington, DC: National Center for Health Statistics.

Guralnik, J. M., & Kaplan, G. A. (1989). Predictors of healthy aging: Prospective evidence from The Alameda County Study. *American Journal of Public Health, 79,* 731–734.

Harrel, F. E. (1980). The logist procedure. In *SAS supplemental library user's guide.* Cary, NC: SAS Institute.

Heyman, A., Tyroler, H. A., Cassel, J. C., O'Fallon, W. M., Davis, L., & Muhlbaier, L. (1976). Geographic differences in mortality from stroke in North Carolina. I. Analysis of death certificates. *Stroke, 7,* 41–45.

House, J. S., Kessler, R., Herzog, A. R., Mero, R. P., Kinney, A. M., & Breslow, M. J. (1989, October). *Social stratification, age and health.* Paper presented at Pennsylvania State Gerontology Center Conference on Aging Health Behaviors, and Health Outcomes, University Park, PA.

Jackson, J. S. (1988). Growing old in black America: Research on aging black populations. In J. S. Jackson (Ed.), *The black American elderly: Research on physical and psychosocial health* (pp. 3–16). New York: Springer.

James, S. A., Wagner, E. H., Strogatz, D. S., Beresford, S. A., Kleinbaum, D. G., Williams, C. A., Cutchin, L. M., & Ibrahim, M. A. (1984). The Edgecombe County High Blood Pressure Control Program: II. Barriers to the use of medical care. *American Journal of Public Health, 74,* 468–472.

James, S. A. (1987a). Psychosocial precursors of hypertension: A review of the epidemiologic evidence. *Circulation, 76*(1), I-60–I-66.

James, S. A., Strogatz, D. S., Wing, S. B., & Ramsey, D. (1987b). Socioeconomic status, John Henryism, and hypertension in blacks and whites. *American Journal of Epidemiology, 126,* 664–673.

Kleinbaum, D. G., Kupper, L. L., & Morgenstern, H. (1982). *Epidemiologic research: Principles and quantitative methods.* Belmont, CA: Lifetime Learning.

Kumanyika, S. (1987). Obesity in black women. *Epidemiologic Reviews, 9*, 31–50.

Liberatos, P., Link, B. G., & Kelsey, J. L. (1988). The measurement of social class in epidemiology. *Epidemiologic Reviews, 10*, 87–121.

Lubben, J. E., Weiler, P. G., & Chi, I. (1989). Health practices of the elderly poor. *American Journal of Public Health, 79*, 731–734.

National Institutes of Health Consensus Development Panel on the Health Implications of Obesity. (1985). Health implications of obesity. *Annals of Internal Medicine, 103*, 983–988.

O'Hare, W. P. (1987). Black demographic trends in the 1980s. *The Milbank Quarterly, 65*(1), 35–55.

Obrist, P. A. (1981). *Cardiovascular psychophysiology: A perspective.* New York: Plenum Press.

Rowe, J. W., & Kahn, R. L. (1987). Human aging: Usual and successful. *Science, 237*, 143–149.

Sempos, C., Cooper, R., Kovar, M. G., & McMiller, M. (1988). Divergence of the recent trends in coronary mortality for the four major race-sex groups in the United States. *American Journal of Public Health, 78*, 1422–1427.

Strogatz, D. S., & James, S. A. (1986). Social support and hypertension among blacks and whites in a rural, southern community. *American Journal of Epidemiology, 124*, 949–956.

Wagner, E. H., James, S. A., Beresford, S. A., Strogatz, D. S., Grimson, R. C., Kleinbaum, D. G., Williams, C. A., Cutchin, L. M., & Ibrahim, M. A. (1984). The Edgecombe County High Blood Pressure Control Program: I. Correlates of uncontrolled hypertension at baseline. *American Journal of Public Health, 74*, 237–242.

Ware, J. E. Jr., Davies-Avery, A., & Donald, C. A. (1978). Conceptualization and measurement of health for adults in the health insurance study. In *General Health Perceptives* (Vol. 5). Santa Monica, CA: Rand Corporation.

Wing, S. B. (1988). Social inequalities in the decline of coronary mortality. *American Journal of Public Health, 78*, 1415–1416.

Social Structure and the Health Behaviors of Blacks

David R. Williams
Yale University

Health behaviors appear to be central determinants of health status. The U.S. Surgeon General, for example, has indicated that almost half of U.S. mortality is attributable to unhealthy behavior or lifestyle (U.S. Department of Health, Education and Welfare, 1979). In comparison, 20% is due to environmental factors, 20% to genetic factors, and 10% to inadequate medical care. It has been estimated that the health status improvements possible through increases in healthy behaviors exceed those that would be achieved if an overnight cure were found for heart disease or cancer (Olshansky, 1985). Moreover, health behaviors are primary determinants of the heavy burden of disease in the Black population. The recent report on Black and Minority Health identified six causes of death that are responsible for 80% of the 60,000 annual excess deaths in the Black (or African-American) population (U.S. Department of Health and Human Services, 1985). Table 1 indicates that cigarette smoking and/or alcohol abuse is a risk factor for five of the six causes of death. Dr. James' insightful and informative chapter highlights the need for more systematic efforts to understand the factors responsible for the social distribution of health behaviors.

The chapter by James et al. also provides unique glimpses into the heterogeneity of the Black population. Much of the research on the health status of African-Americans has utilized a race-comparison paradigm in which the health status of Blacks is compared to that of Whites. Although this research strategy has yielded important information, much research on Blacks continues to compare them to Whites in a routine, mechanical, and atheoretical manner (Gary & Howard, 1979). This comparative approach masks the heterogeneity of the African-American population and fails to identify subgroups that may be especially disadvantaged.

TABLE 1
The Leading Causes of Death for Blacks
and Their Associated Risk Factors

Causes of Death	Risk Factors
Cardiovascular disease	Smoking, high blood pressure, elevated serum cholestrol, obesity, diabetes, lack of exercise.
Cancers	Smoking, alcohol, solar radiation, worksite hazards, environmental contaminants, diet, infectious agents.
Homicide, suicide, and unintentional injuries	Alcohol or drug misuse, stress, handgun availability.
Diabetes	Obesity.
Infant mortality	Low birth weight, maternal smoking, nutrition, stress, trimester of first care, age, marital status.
Cirrhosis of liver	Alcohol.

Source: DHHS (1985).

A central finding of James et al.'s research is that, for both Blacks and Whites, the prevalence of unhealthy behavior is higher among the less educated than among their peers of higher social status. This pattern of results is consistent with national data. Cigarette smoking, for example, is becoming increasingly concentrated among the socioeconomically disadvantaged (Pierce, Fiore, Novotny, Hatziandreau, & Davis, 1989). People with more education are both more likely to quit and less likely to start than their peers with less education. Between 1974 and 1985, for example, the prevalence of smoking declined five times faster among college graduates than among persons with less than a high school education (Pierce et al., 1989). Not surprisingly, smoking rates among Blacks (especially Black males) are higher than among Whites.

This represents a dramatic historic shift in the social distribution of health behaviors. In the 1930s lung cancer death rates for Blacks were half that of Whites, and up through the 1950s smoking rates for Blacks were lower than for Whites (Cooper & Simmons, 1985). Similarly, if we use death rates for cirrhosis of the liver as an indicator of alcohol use, higher levels of alcohol abuse among Blacks than among Whites are also a relatively recent phenomenon. Up though 1955 age-adjusted mortality rates for cirrhosis of the liver were higher for Whites than for Blacks (DHHS, 1985). Accordingly, efforts to understand and address the health problems of the Black population must come to grips with the social structures and processes that facilitate the initiation and maintenance of particular health behaviors.

The mass migration of Blacks from the rural South to the urban North may have played an important role in health behavior changes in the Black population (Cooper & Simmons, 1985). It is likely that several other factors were involved and research that seeks to delineate them would enhance our understanding of the social production of ill health. The critical point is that the behavior of social groups is embedded in their particular social circumstances.

Social structures create stressful living conditions and working environments and shape the adaptive response of social groups. Health behaviors that may have long-term adverse consequences for health status, do provide immediate physiological, psychological, and social benefits that may be necessary for daily survival.

Cigarettes, for example, are widely used as an aid to cope with stress. As Mausner (1973) noted, they "make it possible to get up and face the world, to calm down when tension becomes too great to bear. They take the edge off boring, repetitive tasks like driving, typing and tending machines" (p. 124). A study by the American Cancer Society found that one third of Blacks smoke in order to relieve tension; half of the Black smokers said that smoking was very enjoyable, with an additional one third indicating that it was fairly enjoyable (DHHS, 1985). Moreover, Blacks were more interested in giving up smoking than Whites and were more likely that Whites to believe that quitting would not be difficult. In reality, however, Blacks are less likely than Whites to quit smoking (cf. Fiore et al., 1989). This discrepancy probably reflects both the addictive power of nicotine (Garner, 1986), and the extent to which personal choice is constrained by one's position in social structure.

Understanding the social forces that are linked to the distribution of health behaviors also requires systematic analysis of the targeting of vulnerable populations by large-scale economic interests. Several researchers have noted that women, teenagers, the poor, and members of minority groups are special targets of the tobacco and alcohol industries (Davis, 1987; Singer, 1986). One of the best illustrations of the targeting of a specific group is the detailed description by Hacker, Collins, and Jacobson (1987) of the promotion of alcoholic beverages in the African-American community. The alcohol industry has inextricably tied their products to Black culture. The promotion of alcohol is associated with the music, sports, and cultural events that are integral to the values and tastes of Blacks. Image advertisements in the Black media promote education, fatherhood, Black history, and Black culture. Black celebrities employed by the alcohol industry to promote their products to Blacks include Alex Haley, Wilt Chamberlain, and Lou Rawls. In addition to providing substantial support to Black History Month and the United Negro College Fund, the alcohol industry sponsors an extensive assortment of social, religious, educational, athletic, and business programs for Blacks.

Malt liquors (beer with higher alcohol content) are marketed almost exclusively to Blacks. And the saturation level of alcohol advertising in the Black community is higher than in the predominantly White market. This is evident both in the advertising in the major Black magazines and in the outdoor media. Seventy percent of the eight-sheet billboards in the U.S. contain advertisements targeted to Blacks. Cigarettes are the number one product advertised on the medium and alcohol is number two. Moreover, some alcohol producers link economic support of the Black community to increased sales of the company's products; and enlist the support of community leaders toward this end. For example, when the Adolph Coors Co. agreed to invest $625 million over 5 years in Black and Hispanic areas, the NAACP, Operation PUSH, and the African Methodist Episcopal Church's Western District, among others, agreed to "take positive visible action to help eliminate the misconceptions of Coors" (Hacker et al., 1987, p. 34).

In addition to the ubiquitous presence of commercial enticement, alcoholic beverages are also more readily available to the poor and minorities. Retail outlets for alcohol are more prevalent in low income and minority neighborhoods than in more affluent communities (Rabow & Watt, 1982). And there is a strong positive relationship between the availability of alcohol and the amount of alcohol consumption (Singer, 1986).

I concur with James et al. that the high prevalence of cigarette smoking in the youngest age groups is especially disturbing. However, it is not surprising given the extent to which teenagers are currently being targeted by the tobacco industry (Davis, 1987; Journal of the American Medical Association, 1986). The tobacco interests are well aware that 95% of adult smokers started smoking between the ages of 12 and 21 (Arbogast, 1986). In fact, 85% of adolescents who smoke more than one cigarette will become long-term smokers (Garner, 1986). And the tobacco industry's message that associates smoking with youth, health, romance, adventure,and success is frequently the only one that teenagers hear. The annual budget of the Office of Smoking and Health (OSH) is equivalent to the daily budget of the tobacco advertisers (Arbogast, 1986) and the annual spending on smoking deterrence activities of the OSH and the three major voluntary health organizations amounts to only 1% of the advertising expenditures of the tobacco industry (Gitlitz, 1983).

The James et al. data also indicated that the prevalence of smoking was relatively low among Black females, clearly indicating that high rates of smoking are not uniform in disadvantaged populations. This finding also suggests that attempts to identify social structures that facilitate the initiation of unhealthy behaviors must include efforts to identify countervailing forces. Other data indicate that Black females also have high rates of abstention from alcohol. It is likely that the high level of religious involvement in this population may be linked to the observed patterns of substance use. More systematic efforts to understand and facilitate the health-promoting efforts of the Black church are clearly warranted.

The high prevalence of obesity in middle-aged African-American females was also evident in the Edgecombe County data. Some of my own research, using data from the National Health and Nutrition Examination Survey, indicates that the higher prevalence of obesity in Black females, as compared to their White peers, can completely explain race differences in systolic and diastolic blood pressure (Williams & Bryant, 1989). These findings highlight the urgency of James et al.'s call for "detailed studies of environmental, behavioral and biologic risk factors for obesity in black women.'' It is likely that physical inactivity among Black females makes an important contribution to the high rate of obesity. Given that most exercise is obtained through leisure-time physical activity, research efforts must address the degree to which African-American females lack the opportunities and resources, economic and otherwise, to engage in regular physical exercise. Another promising direction for research is the exploration of the extent to which recurrent eating binges, associated with the use of food to gain comfort and relief from stress, contributes to obesity in Black females (Williams, in press).

Finally, taking seriously the role that large-scale social structures and processes have on the creation of the social distribution of health behavior, in particular, and a broad range of psychosocial factors more generally, has implications for the way we do research. Health enhancing and health damaging resources cannot be viewed as autonomous individual factors, unrelated to living and working conditions and independent of the broader social and political order. Renewed attention must be given to identifying why populations, as opposed to individuals, vary in their level of risk factors. Studies of the characteristics of populations can facilitate the specification of large-scale processes that affect the production of ill heath.

Researchers must also give more explicit attention to the social, economic, and political forces that constrain the lives of participants in their research studies. Much research on health behaviors and risk factors focuses narrowly on selected aspects of people's lives without attending to ways in which both subjective reality and objective conditions of life are shaped by socioeconomic position. The collection of survey research data in a community study, for example, should be combined with an understanding of the social and economic structure of that community and the ways in which these conditions shape the values and behavior of social groups.

Nicholas Dorn's (1980) study of alcohol use among teenagers entering the job market is an excellent example of the kind of research that is needed. In addition to interviewing teenagers, Dorn (1980) also conducted interviews with guidance counselors and teachers, and studied the local labor market by researching documentary evidence, interviewing local employers, and visiting local workplaces. He was thus able to identify the ways in which socioeconomic position and occupational conditions shaped the daily realities and experiences of teenagers and gave rise to distinctive patterns of alcohol use. Research that fails to seriously address the social origins of illness, will serve to maintain the status quo and perpetuate the already widespread distortion of social reality.

ACKNOWLEDGMENT

Preparation of this chapter was supported by grant AG-07904 from the National Institute of Aging.

REFERENCES

Arbogast, R. (1986). A proposal to regulate the manner of tobacco advertising. *Journal of Health Politics, Policy and Law, 11*, 393–422.

Cooper, R. & Simmons, B. E (1985). Cigarette smoking and ill heath among black Americans. *New York State Journal of Medicine, 85*, 344–349.

Davis, R. M. (1987). Current trends in cigarette advertising and marketing. *New England Journal of Medicine, 316*, 725–732.

Dorn, N. (1980). Alcohol in teenage cultures: A materialist approach to youth cultures, drinking and health education. *Health Education Journal, 39*, 67–73.

Fiore, M. C., Novotny, T., Pierce, J., Hatziandreau, E., Patel, K., & Davis, R. (1989). Trends in cigarette smoking in the United States: The changing influence of gender and race. *Journal of the American Medical Association, 261*, 49–55.

Garner, D. W. (1986). Tobacco sampling, public policy and the law. *Journal of Health Politics, Policy and Law, 11*, 423–443.

Gary, L., & Howard, C. (1979). Policy implications of mental health research for Black Americans. *Urban League Review 4*, 16–24.

Gitlitz, G. (1983). Cigarette advertising and the New York Times: An ethical issue that's unfit to print? *New York State Journal of Medicine, 83*, 1284–1291.

Hacker, A., Collins, R., & Jacobson, M. (1987). *Marketing booze to Blacks*. Washington, DC: Center for Science in the Public Interest.

Journal of the American Medical Association. (1986). Alcohol: Advertising, counteradvertising, and depiction in the public media. *JAMA, 256*, 1485–1488.

Mausner, B. (1973). An ecological view of cigarette smoking. *Journal of Abnormal Psychology, 81*, 115–126.

Olshansky, S. J. (1985). Pursuing longevity: Delay vs. elimination of degenerative diseases. *American Journal of Public Health, 75*, 754–757.

Pierce, J. P., Fiore, M., Novotny, T. E., Hatziandreau, E., & Davis, R. (1989). Trends in cigarette smoking in the United States: Educational differences are increasing. *Journal of the American Medical Association, 261*, 56–65.

Rabow, J., & Watt, R. (1982). Alcohol availability, alcohol beverage sales and alcohol-related problems. *Journal of Studies on Alcohol, 43*, 767–801.

Singer, M. (1986). Toward a political economy of alcoholism. *Social Science and Medicine, 23*, 113–130.

U.S. Department of Health, Education and Welfare. (1979). *Healthy People: The Surgeon General's Report on Health Promotion and Disease Prevention*. Washington, DC: United States Government Printing Office.

U.S. Department of Health and Human Services. (1985). *Report of the Secretary's Task Force on Black and Minority Health*. Washington, DC: United States Government Printing Office.

Williams, D. R. (in press). Race, social structure, and high blood pressure. In W. Davis & G. King (Eds.), *The health of black America: Social causes and consequences*. Oxford: Oxford University Press.

Williams, D. R., & Bryant, S. (1989). Race differences in hypertension: Identifying the determinants. In *Proceedings of the 1989 Public Health Conference on Records and Statistics* (DHHS Pub. No. (PHS) 90-1214, pp. 422–427). Washington, DC: U.S. Government Printing Office.

Discussion of Socioeconomic Status, Health Behaviors, and Health Status Among Blacks

George L. Maddox
Duke University

The James et al. chapter, along with the chapter by House et al. preceding it, illustrates the strengths and limitations of contemporary social epidemiology. The specific substantive focus of the chapter by James and his colleagues on how the social location of Blacks might affect health behavior and health status is timely and important. The prose and argument are clear. The authors are aware of their limited generalizability. The data are cross-sectional and the inability of the authors to address age, period, and cohort issues and the dynamics of interactions of individuals and milieus as they affect health is acknowledged. The small size of the sample reduces the utility of multivariate analyses.

Substantively the investigators report no unexpected results. Blacks and Whites are different in health status and health behaviors and higher socioeconomic status (SES) predicts healthful behavior and outcomes. That said, one can concentrate on several important theoretical and methodological issues illustrated in the chapter. Of particular interest to me are the chapter's illustration of some strengths and weaknesses of social epidemiological inquiry such as the de-emphasis of direct measurement of social context in social survey research procedures adopted by social epidemiologists; problems of conceptualizing and describing developmental processes in the analysis of cross-sectional data; and the relevance of epidemiological risk analysis for health policy.

THE THOUGHTSTYLE OF SOCIAL EPIDEMIOLOGY

Social epidemiology is the offspring of classical epidemiology as a branch of medicine and of social survey technology. I was a post-doctoral fellow at the University of London in the late 1960s when Jerome Morris arrived as the new dean of the School of Hygiene and Tropical Medicine. He had new ideas about epidemiology and its uses which, as outlined in his *Uses of Epidemiology* (1967), included a broadening of the concept of noxious agents to include sociological variables and a rationale for why physician-epidemiologists should learn social survey technology, sampling design, and computerization of data. Not every student of this new epidemiology was equally enthusiastic about what appeared to be the possible substitution for clinical assessment of measuring health by self-report or other proxy measures. In the United States, social epidemiology became the domain of social scientists interested in health and health care who in survey research using large samples seemed comfortable with using self-reports of health, disease, and behavioral risk factors. Contacts between social epidemiologists and physicians have become substantially attenuated.

James and his co-authors are social epidemiologists who do not include any clinical material in their study. They explore in their small, geographically bounded sample three health outcomes (hypertension, obesity, and self-rated health) and two health behaviors (cigarette smoking and physical exercise). From the perspective of a medical clinician, this may appear as truncated although clearly specified conceptualization of health status and health behaviors to which the chapter's title refers.

Both classical and social epidemiology continued to share an interest in SES as one of the most persistently powerful predictors of risk factors, morbidity and mortality. The happenstance of sampling design that limited the measurement of social status to education (years of schooling) in this research nonetheless made an important point. Years of schooling completed is increasingly recognized in epidemiology as an independent predictor of health behavior and status whose effect is not adequately accounted for by income alone. This conclusion is illustrated once again. Risk factors, perceived health status perception, and hypertension tend, for both Blacks and Whites, to be negatively associated with education.

An epidemiological thoughtstyle historically has featured the measurement of the physical and social contexts in which health behavior and health outcomes develop. Social epidemiologists, when embracing strategies of social survey research, have attenuated significantly their ability to measure the proximate environment directly.

LEAVING OUT MILIEU

Getting the benefits of social survey technology in social epidemiology has exacted a price and, in my view, a considerable price. Emphasis on probability samples representing large, geographically dispersed populations has tended to make the location of individuals in a measured social milieu impractical if not impossible. Social surveyors and social epidemiologists have tended to set-tle for self-reports of individuals about the social contexts (communities, neigh-borhoods, workplaces) in which they live and work. Social epidemiology fo-cuses on individuals, not milieus. Figure 1 illustrates particularly well a useful distinction between microscopic (individual) variables in research and macro-scopic (societal) variables relevant to the assertion that social epidemiologists frequently if not typically neglect contextual variables.

Contemporary social survey research has tended to declare its disinterest in, or its inability to be seriously interested in, locating individuals in social and societal contexts. This is not all bad; individuals per se warrant study. But it is consequential for interpreting findings and assessing causal explana-tions to study only individuals. In particular, the social, as distinct from the biological meaning of race in the research of James and his colleagues, is difficult to interpret without reference to the dynamics of race relationships and to the allocation of resources and opportunities in the community in which the study subjects have lived and worked. More generally, one notes that the authors study individuals in a community and not the community. Absence of infor-mation about the community would also be consequential for any discussion about practical interventions intended to improve health behaviors or health status among Blacks. The authors do find, as one might anticipate, that edu-cation differentiates some but not all health behaviors and outcomes for both Whites and Blacks. Quite commonly, White/Black differences disappear as soon as control is introduced for income, a test not possible in this particular study.

AGE, PERIOD, AND COHORT

The authors acknowledge that one cannot equate age differences and age changes. They acknowledge that age changes may be period-specific and cohort-specific. This cross-sectional research does not and cannot explore this issue.

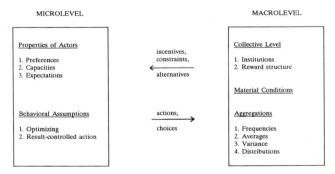

FIG. 1. The dynamic relationship between microlevel and macrolevel vari-ables in the study of human aging (*Source*: Maddox & Campbell, 1985).

The reader is forewarned. One might wish, then, that the data presentation on the relation of age to health behaviors and outcomes were different. A false inference is invited when age differences observed in variables of interest are presented as though they are regression lines with definitive age-related slopes. This is not what the authors intend to convey regarding the representation of age differences. Bar graphs, however, would be more appropriate in making clear the data represent cross-sectional age differences, not age changes. The authors appropriately call for future research appropriate for addressing more definitively age, period, cohort differences among Blacks.

PUBLIC INVESTMENT TO IMPROVE HEALTH

Historically, classical epidemiology shared with medicine generally a clinical interest in identifying risks and negative outcomes in order to guide corrective interventions. It is my impression that this traditional clinical imperative in classical epidemiology to anticipate interventions is not as commonly observed in social epidemiology. In any case, it is not observed in the report of James and his associates. On the other hand, Chapter 1 by House and colleagues, concludes with some rather strong specific recommendations regarding the social policy implications of their finding that income and education are powerful predictors of health and functional status. The remedy for age-related poor health and impairment is not "consider seeing your doctor and visit your hospital" but "consider a differential distribution of economic and educational resources." The appeal in this case is not to individuals action but to changing political institutions and societal values (see Fig. 1). Following this advice would be facilitated by knowing more about the societal variables (Fig. 1) that characterize the milieus in which individuals live and work and in demonstrating how the societal rather than just the biological variables produce differences in healthy lifestyles and healthy outcomes. Consequently, one might wish for more interest in the measurement of environments than is characteristic of a great deal of contemporary social epidemiology in the interest both of understanding and improving health.

REFERENCES

Maddox, G., & Campbell, R. (1985). Scope, concepts, and methods in the study of aging. In R. Binstock & E. Shanas (Eds.), *Handbook of aging and the social sciences* (pp. 3–34). New York: Van Nostrand Reinhold.
Morris, J. (1967). *Uses of epidemiology* (2nd ed.). London: S. & S. Livingstone.

Health and Aging
in the Alameda County Study

George A. Kaplan
Human Population Laboratory, Berkeley, CA

INTRODUCTION

It is only relatively recently that the aging process and its relationship to health has attracted the interest of epidemiologists. The impact of age on the health outcomes that have become so prevalent during the last half century is so strong, that it became common to simply include age in all analyses as an adjustment variable. Although this strategy permitted public health researchers to get on with many important tasks, including the development of the preventive approaches that have been so successful, it led to a pervasive lack of knowledge concerning the relationships between aging and health.

The increasingly important changes in the age structure of the United States, and most industrialized countries have, fortunately, led to a revaluation of this perspective, and an explosion of research in the epidemiology of aging. Based on the new evidence, there are several evolving view points that need to be emphasized. First, there is now a general recognition that the elderly of today are different from those of the past. In addition to occupying a substantially greater proportion of the population, today's elderly differ on a wide variety of demographic, social, and behavioral dimensions from those of earlier generations (Riley, 1981). Critical comparative issues concerning the health of the elderly, the discussion of the compression of morbidity, are being hotly debated (Fries, 1980, 1983, 1984; Manton, 1982; Schneider & Brody, 1983; Schneider & Guralnik, 1987). Second, a growing literature documents the importance of not confusing disease with aging. Chronic, degenerative diseases are now being seen as separate from aging, and not a necessary result of aging (Rowe & Kahn, 1987). Third, the wide variations, with aging, in health trajectories and outcomes suggest that there may be distinctly different pathways of aging, and there is an increasing recognition of the need to acknowledge this enormous variability (Manton & Soldo, 1985; Rowe & Kahn, 1987). Finally, at the same time as there is increasing interest in the physiology and molecular biology of aging, there is a growing appreciation of the need to study aging within a broad perspective that includes behavioral, social, demographic, psychological, and other factors (Kaplan & Haan, 1989; Kaplan, Seeman, Cohen, Knudsen, & Guralnik, 1987; Lazarus, Kaplan, Cohen, & Leu, 1989; Rowe & Kahn, 1987; Seeman, Kaplan, Knudsen, Cohen, & Guralnik, 1987).

It is important not to lose sight of the steep increases with age in the prevalence and toll from many diseases. For example, Fig. 3.1 shows the exponential increases in death rates that occur with increasing age (National Center for Health Statistics, 1988). Similar increases are seen for most of the morbidities that exact the biggest population burden. Given the rapid rise in morbidity that is coincident with increasing age, and the large increases in life expectancy at the older ages (Brody, Dwight, & Williams, 1987), it is of great importance to know if preventive efforts might be efficacious for older persons (Kaplan & Haan, 1989).

Epidemiologic approaches to prevention have, generally, started with the identification of associations between risk factors and health outcomes, leading ultimately to interventions directed at preventing, removing, or lowering the levels of these risk factors. However, the examination of such associations in older persons has been influenced by several beliefs. It has long been believed that persons who survive to older ages represent a select group of the

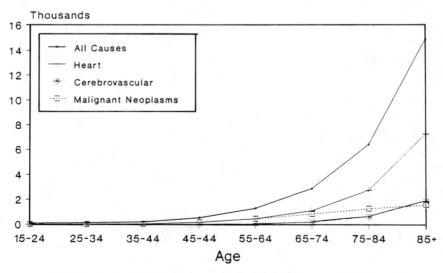

FIG. 3.1. Annual mortality rates (per 100,000) for all causes and selected causes and selected causes by age, United States, 1984.

population for whom a specific risk factor might have been relatively unimportant. For example, from this perspective tobacco exposure should not matter for a person aged 70 or older because those who were truly susceptible to the impact of tobacco exposure would already have suffered premature deaths from heart disease or lung cancer. Also, given the cumulative effects of exposure to risk factors, it was felt that changes late in life could not reverse the damage that had already been caused by smoking or other risk factors. Early studies indicating that risk factor effects declined at the older ages generally supported such views (Kannel & Gordon, 1980).

Although those who survive to older ages undoubtedly reflect a selected population, the impact of this selection is complex (Vaupel & Yashin, 1985), and does not guarantee that risk factor effects will be negligible at older ages. The impact of these selection factors is real, however, it needs to be emphasized that most chronic diseases are multifactorial in nature, with no one risk factor accounting for the bulk of the disease experience. Furthermore, even if the association between a risk factor and a health outcome decreases somewhat among older persons, the greatly increased risk of the outcome in that group means that the risk factor can still have a significant population burden of compromised health. Finally, for reasons that are not entirely clear, the majority of recent studies differ from the earlier studies in that they have indicated a substantial role for behavioral, social, demographic, and, to a limited extent, psychological risk factors in the health of older persons.

In what follows, we examine this latter point in some detail using data collected as part of the Alameda County Study, a large-scale prospective study of adult residents of a typical urban county that was initiated in 1965 by the Human Population Laboratory of the California Department of Health Services (Berkman & Breslow, 1983; Hochstim, 1970). Unlike many of the population-based studies initiated around that time, the 1965 Alameda County Study had no upward restrictions on age. The result was a baseline sample that numbered almost 7,000, with an age range of 16–94 years. These respondents have been followed up on two occasions, 1974 and 1983, and their mortality and cancer morbidity experience has been monitored continuously since the study's inception.

DETERMINANTS OF MORTALITY FROM ALL CAUSES

Health Status

Because most of the causes of death among older persons represent the consequences of cumulative disease processes, it is not surprising that chronic conditions and symptoms reported by Alameda County Study respondents are strongly associated with subsequent risk of death. For those who were 60–94 years old in 1965, the self-reports of heart trouble, high blood pressure, diabetes, chest pain, or shortness of breath were associated with a 45%–60% increased risk of death, compared to those without the particular conditions, over the next 19 years. Those 45% who reported all five conditions and symptoms were at a three-fold risk of death (Relative Hazard = 3.00, 95% Confidence Interval, 2.68-3.35) compared to the 55% who reported none. In other analyses, those with 3 or more conditions and symptoms out of a list of 22, were at 1.24-fold increased risk of death (95% Confidence Interval, 1.03-1.49) compared to those who reported none (Seeman, Guralnik, Kaplan, Knudsen, & Cohen, 1989). Global perception of health status, perceived health, was also strongly associated with risk of death. Over a 9-year follow-up period, men and women over 60 years old who reported that their health was "poor" were at 1.52 and 2.82-fold increased risk of death, respectively, compared to those who reported their health "excellent" (Kaplan & Camacho, 1983). This increased risk was independent of other measures of physical health status, health practices, social network participation, and other covariables.

Behavioral Factors

A number of behaviorally-related factors have been identified as strong determinants of mortality risk in older Alameda County Study participants. Figure 3.2 presents the results of these analyses for those 70 years or more old who were followed for mortality over a 17-year period (Kaplan et al., 1987). Even among those who had survived until age 70, smoking continues to exact a significant toll. With adjustment for age, sex, baseline health status, and other significant predictors, those who were current smokers had 1.43 times (95% Confidence Interval, 1.08-1.89) the risk of death of those who were never smokers. Past smokers did not differ significantly from never smokers (Relative Risk = 1.01, 95% Confidence Interval, 0.76-1.33). In additional analyses, quitting smoking was shown to have a significant protective effect on subsequent mortality (Kaplan & Haan, 1989). Among those 50–94 years old in 1965, the risk of subsequent death for those who quit smoking between the 1965 baseline interview and a follow-up interview in 1974 was considerably different from those who continued smoking. Compared to never smokers, 1965–1974 quitters were at 33% increased risk (Relative Hazard = 1.33, 95% Confidence Interval, 0.98-1.82), whereas those who continued smoking were at 76% increased risk (Relative Hazard = 1.76, 95% Confidence Interval, 1.35-2.31). Those who quit before the baseline interview did not differ from those who never smoked (Relative Hazard = 1.06, 95% Confidence Interval, 0.79-1.42).

Physical activity and changes in level of physical activity were importantly associated with mortality risk among older respondents in the Alameda County Study. In analyses examining the 17-year mortality risk of respondents 70–94

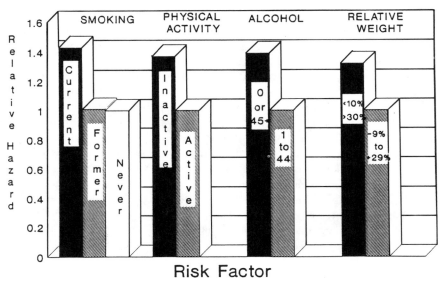

Alameda County Study

FIG. 3.2. Association between behavioral risk factors and 17-year risk of death in those 70–94 years.

years old, physical inactivity was associated with a 37% increased risk of death (Relative Hazard = 1.37, 95% Confidence Interval, 1.09-1.72), with adjustment for age, physical health status, smoking, and relative weight (Kaplan et al., 1987). Interestingly, this increased risk associated with physical inactivity varied very little from that for the younger respondents. Changes in level of physical activity were also importantly related to subsequent risk of death (Kaplan & Haan, 1989). Respondents aged 50–94 who increased their level of physical activity were at significantly decreased risk compared to those who maintained the same level, and those who decreased their level of activity were at significantly increased risk. This impact of change in physical activity level on subsequent risk of death was maintained in analyses restricted to those who were healthy at baseline, and were independent of incident chronic conditions, alcohol consumption, smoking changes, weight changes, and body mass index.

Alcohol consumption is also related to risk among the older members of the Alameda County Study, with those who abstained or consumed more than 45 drinks per month at increased risk compared to those who consumed 1–25 drinks per month (Kaplan et al., 1987). In this case the increased risk was 39% for the first two groups compared to the moderate drinkers (Relative Hazard = 1.39, 95% Confidence Interval, 0.94-2.05). Analyses of the association between changes in alcohol consumption and subsequent risk of death, currently underway, suggest that the increased risk among abstainers is due primarily to those who are former drinkers but who stopped drinking. The presumption being that the change in drinking habits was associated with health status changes (Lazarus, Kaplan, & Cohen, 1991).

Relative weight, which is partially influenced by behavioral factors, was also related to risk of death. For those 70–94, being more than 10% underweight or 30% overweight was associated with a 32% increased risk (Relative Hazard = 1.32, 95% Confidence Interval, 1.05-1.67) compared to those of moderate weight (Kaplan et al., 1987). Changes in weight, for those 50–94 years old, were also associated with risk of death (Kaplan & Haan, 1989). The main increased risk was associated with decreases in weight, with a 14-pound decline over a 9-year period resulting in a 48% increased risk of death compared to those who maintained the same weight (Relative Hazard = 1.48, 95% Confidence Interval, 1.18-1.85). These results, which have been confirmed in other studies, suggest that unintentional weight loss among the elderly is cause for concern.

Social Factors

Figure 3.3 illustrates the association between a number of measures of social connections and mortality risk in Alameda County Study respondents 70–94 years old in 1965 (Seeman et al., 1987). Being unmarried, which at younger ages is associated with increased risk in this cohort, is no longer so associated in those over 70 years old (Relative Hazard = 1.15, 95% Confidence Interval, 0.93-1.43). On the other hand, those who reported fewer than five close friends or relatives seen at least once per month, labeled socially isolated, were at 31% higher risk (Relative Hazard = 1.31, 95% Confidence Interval, 1.05-1.62) than those who reported a greater number of contacts. Non-membership in church groups and in other types of groups were both associated with increased risk (Relative Hazard = 1.32, 95% Confidence Interval, 1.08-1.62 and Relative Hazard = 1.20, 95% Confidence Interval, 0.99-1.46, respectively). A summary measure of social network participation, the Social Network Index (Berkman & Breslow, 1983), was also strongly associated with risk of death in those over 70 years old. Those who were in the lowest category of the index had a mortality risk that was 1.69 times higher (95% Confidence Interval, 1.24-2.29) compared to those in the highest category.

Changes in social contacts are also important predictors of mortality risk in this cohort. Nine-year declines in numbers of close friends, close relatives, number of close friends and relatives seen at least once per month, and total numbers of contacts were all associated with increased risk of death compared to those who did not experience such declines (Kaplan & Haan, 1989), the increased risk ranging from 22% to 77%. These results were independent of

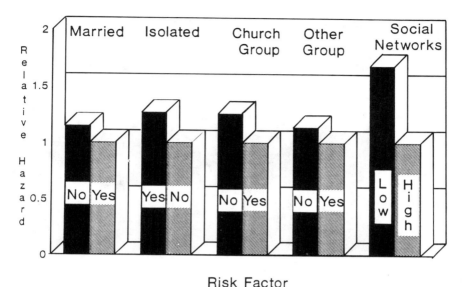

Alameda County Study

FIG. 3.3. Association between social risk factors and 17-year risk of death
in those 70–94 years.

the presence of chronic conditions and symptoms at baseline, incident conditions and symptoms, and other covariables.

Demographic Factors

Figure 3.4 illustrates the relationship between a variety of demographic factors and 17-year risk of death among older participants in the Alameda County Study. The sex difference in mortality, observed in many studies, persists among those 60 years or older and is virtually identical when the analyses involve only those 70 years or older (Kaplan et al., 1987). There is, however, some diminution of the male excess with increasing age, largely due to female rates of cardiovascular disease increasing faster than male rates from age 50 on (Wingard, Cohn, Kaplan, Cirillo, & Cohen, 1989).

A comparison of Black and White mortality rates at this age shows that the Black disadvantage at earlier ages has been eliminated and, perhaps, even reversed (Kaplan et al., 1987). For those who were 60 years old or more in 1965, Blacks were at slightly lower risk over the next 17 years (Relative Hazard = 0.93, 95% Confidence Interval, 0.70-1.22). This "crossover" effect, which has been found in other analyses is not well understood, and may reflect

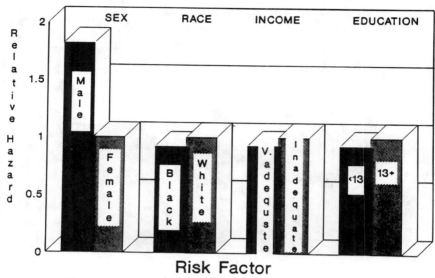

FIG. 3.4. Association between demographic risk factors and 17-year risk of death in those 70–94 years.

the combined effect of differential survivorship and risk factor exposure, cohort effects, and misreporting of age.

Measures of socioeconomic position, education and income, are no longer associated with mortality risk in older persons in the Alameda County Study. When the association between income and 17-year mortality was examined for those 60 years or older, those in the bottom quintile of the distribution of family income adjusted for family size were not at increased risk compared to those in the top quintile (Relative Hazard = 0.90, 95% Confidence Interval, 0.71-1.14). This was in contrast with a much stronger association for those 38–59 years old (Relative Hazard = 1.73, 95% Confidence Interval, 1.29-2.31). Similar results were found when the association between level of education and 17-year risk of death was examined. Those who were over 60 years old in 1965 and had more than a high school education were actually at somewhat higher, but not significant, risk compared to those with less education (Relative Hazard = 1.14, 95% Confidence Interval, 0.91-1.43). For those who were 38–59 years old, there was a considerably elevated risk associated with lower education (Relative Hazard = 1.34, 95% Confidence Interval, 0.96-1.87). The lack of an association between level of income and risk of death probably reflects the fact that it is not a good measure of the economic resources of older persons, whereas the absence of an association with education may reflect cohort differences.

Socioenvironmental factors are also related to mortality risk among older respondents in the Alameda County Study. In an analysis of the cohort members who lived in Oakland, California, the largest city in Alameda County, the association between residence in federally designated poverty areas and mortality was examined (Haan, Kaplan, & Camacho, 1987). For those who were 55 years old or more, residence in such areas was associated with 26% higher 9-year mortality risk when compared to those who did not live in such areas (95% Confidence Interval, 0.96-1.67). What's more, this increased risk persisted when there was adjustment for age, race, gender, income, employment status, access to medical care, health insurance coverage, smoking, physical activity, body mass index, and other risk factors. The analyses were expanded to all of Alameda County, however, instead of using residence in a poverty area as the predictor, a series of scales were developed based on demographic and socioenvironmental characteristics of Alameda County census tracts. Several of these scales were strongly associated with subsequent risk of death among older persons. For example, those 60-year-olds who lived in census tracts that had high proportions of separated or divorced persons, deteriorating housing units, blue-collar workers, and Blacks were at 1.67-fold risk of death over 9 years (95% Confidence Interval, 1.17-2.39) compared to those who lived in census tracts that had low proportions. For another scale that measured the proportion of males older than 65 years, housing units with no bath or shared bath and with no heat, and widowed males, there was also increased risk (Relative Hazard = 1.37, 95% Confidence Interval, 1.06-1.77). These increased risks were maintained even when there was adjustment for the long list of potential confounders used in the poverty area analyses. Thus, there is an indication that socioenvironmental characteristics of the areas in which older people live may be independent predictors of their subsequent health.

Psychological Factors

A number of psychological factors have been shown to be associated with mortality risk in the Alameda County Study (Kaplan, 1985). For example, those who report high levels of depressive symptoms are at higher risk of death compared to those who do not. For those over 60 years of age, high levels of depressive symptoms are associated with a 1.4-fold (95% Confidence Interval, 1.15-1.75) increase in 9-year mortality risk. However, when there is adjustment for the presence of chronic conditions, symptoms, and disability, there is no association (Relative Hazard = 1.08, 95% Confidence Interval, 0.85-1.36). Thus, the relationship between depressive symptoms and all cause mortality among older persons seems to reflect the higher rates of depression among those who are sick (Kaplan & Reynolds, 1988; Roberts, Kaplan, & Camacho, 1990).

Life satisfaction and personal uncertainty, a measure of helplessness (Berkman & Breslow, 1983), are also associated with mortality risk among older persons in the Alameda County Study. Those over 60 years of age who were dissatisfied, were at 1.65 times the 9-year risk of death when compared to those who were not (95% Confidence Interval, 1.24-2.20). Again, however, a good deal of the association appears to be due to higher rates of illness among those who are dissatisfied. With adjustment for chronic conditions, symptoms, and disabilities, the association is considerably weakened (Relative Hazard = 1.32, 95% Confidence Interval, 0.98-1.78). Those who indicated high levels of personal uncertainty were also at increased risk (Relative Hazard = 1.35, 95% Confidence Interval, 1.04-1.75), but this association was not appreciably weakened by adjustment for prevalent illness and disability (Relative Hazard = 1.23, 95% Confidence Interval, 0.94-1.61).

DETERMINANTS OF FUNCTIONAL HEALTH

Death, of course, is not the only outcome of interest in epidemiologic studies of aging and health. The increasing numbers of persons who are surviving to older ages has led many to be concerned with the assessment of functional status. This focus views physical, psychological, and social functioning as critical and interacting dimensions of the health of older persons. A number of analyses have been completed using the Alameda County Study that bear upon this approach. Long-range predictors of physical functioning were studied in a sample of study participants who were at least 65 years old (Guralnik, 1985). In this study, a broad measure of physical functioning was used that enabled respondents to be ordered on a scale ranging from having difficulties with basic activities of daily living to participating in active sports. Predictors were taken from the interview 19 years earlier in 1965 when the respondents were at least 48 years old. Table 3.1 shows the variables that, in multiple regression models,

TABLE 3.1
1965 Predictors of 1984 Functional Health Status
(from Guralnik, 1985)

Variable	Beta	p ( )
Age	− 0.34	.0001
Race	− 4.26	.0005
Health	− 1.82	.04
Disability	− 2.78	.008
Smoking	− 2.22	.006
Weight/height	2.37	.014
Income	1.49	.004
Marital status	3.00	.0014
Physical activity	2.68	.008

TABLE 3.2
Association Between Incident Health Problems
and Incident ADL Problems

	Odds Ratio (95% C.I.) ADL	
	Feeding, dressing, or moving	Climbing stairs or getting outdoors
Stroke	6.61 (3.52,12.39)	6.78 (3.78,12.17)
Heart trouble	2.82 (1.66,4.80)	5.12 (3.40,7.70)
Arthritis	2.14 (1.11,4.10)	2.13 (1.35,3.36)
Diabetes	1.84 (0.76,4.46)	3.23 (1.72,6.04)
Chest pain	2.88 (1.55,5.35)	4.36 (2.71,7.02)
Shortness of breath	4.06 (2.32,7.11)	4.50 (2.85,7.09)
Back pain	2.21 (1.18,4.13)	2.34 (1.50,3.64)
Joint stiffness	4.02 (2.16,7.51)	4.99 (3.28,7.60)

were significantly associated with higher levels of physical functioning 19 years later, when the respondents were 65–89 years old. These predictors cover a broad range, ranging from earlier levels of physical activity and health status to demographic, behavioral, social and psychological domains. Similar results were found when the analyses focused on predictors of high levels of functioning, an aspect of healthy aging (Guralnik & Kaplan, 1989).

In other analyses, in which attention was focused on limitations in the ability to perform activities of daily living, there were similar findings. For example, among those who were 55–94 years of age in 1965, 9-year incidence of limitations in climbing stairs or getting outdoors were higher among those who were current smokers (Odds Ratio = 1.93, 95% Confidence Interval, 1.24-3.01), depressed (Odds Ratio = 2.24, 95% Confidence Interval, 1.36-3.68), or who had inadequate versus very adequate incomes (Odds Ratio = 2.13, 95% Confidence Interval, 1.11-4.12).

The major predictors of difficulties in performing activities of daily living are, of course, related to health problems. Table 3.2 presents the results of analyses that examine the association, in those 50 years old or more, between 1965–1974 incidence of chronic conditions and symptoms and incidence of limitations in activities of daily living in the same period. As can be seen, the associations are very strong. However, above and beyond the influence of chronic conditions and symptoms, there is an impact of behavioral, social, psychological, and demographic factors. Among those who were incident cases of heart trouble, stroke, diabetes, or arthritis, the rates of mobility limitations were higher in those who smoked (Odds Ratio = 2.02, 95% Confidence Interval, 1.21-3.38), who were depressed (Odds Ratio = 1.76, 95% Confidence Interval, 0.95-3.27), who were socially isolated (Odds Ratio = 1.95, 95% Confidence Interval, 0.97-3.91), and who had inadequate incomes (Odds Ratio = 3.54, 95% Confidence Interval, 1.50-8.36).

This pattern of results, in which there are important predictors representing health status, behavioral, social, psychological, and demographic factors is repeated when psychological functioning is considered. Factors predictive of high levels of depressive symptoms have been examined in the Alameda County Study, using a symptom check list similar to the CES-D and the other measures of depressive symptoms that have been used in epidemiologic studies (Kaplan, Roberts, Camacho, & Coyne, 1987). For example, for those over 60 years old in 1965 a number of factors were importantly associated with level of depressive symptoms in 1974, with adjustment for age and level of symptoms at baseline: less than high school education (Odds Ratio = 3.16, 95% Confidence Interval, 1.79-5.61), inadequate income (Odds Ratio = 2.29, 95% Confidence Interval, 1.28-4.10), ADL limitations (Odds Ratio = 3.33, 95% Confidence Interval, 1.42-7.81), chronic conditions (Odds Ratio = 2.11, 95% Confidence Interval, 0.92-4.88), poor versus excellent perceived health (Odds Ratio = 2.96, 95% Confidence Interval, 2.08-4.20), personal uncertainty (Odds Ratio = 1.88, 95% Confidence Interval, 1.07-3.30), loss of a spouse (Odds Ratio = 2.18, Confidence Interval, 1.17-4.07), money stress (Odds Ratio = 2.31, 95% Confidence Interval, 0.95-5.54), and social isolation (Odds Ratio = 1.91, Confidence Interval, 0.88-4.14). Thus, many of the factors that are associated with mortality risk or with levels of physical functioning are also associated with depression.

DETERMINANTS OF RISK FACTOR CHANGE

Older persons, just like younger persons, are not static. Their behaviors, social relationships, feelings, and other characteristics change over time. However, there has been remarkably little attention paid to the patterns of risk factor change over time in older persons, or the factors that contribute to those changes. Because the Alameda County Study interviewed respondents on several occasions it was possible to examine, in a preliminary way, the natural history of risk factor change.

Figure 3.5 presents information on baseline physical activity by age, and the percent change in physical activity level between 1965 and 1974 (Lazarus et al., 1989). A simple measure of leisure-time physical activity, which is related to subsequent mortality risk, based on reports of the frequency of participation in active sports, swimming or taking long walks, working in the garden, and doing physical exercises was used. Generally speaking, levels of physical activity decline with age, more so in women than in men, with a major change occurring after age 60. This age-related decline, however, is not automatic, as there is considerable variability. When the reasons for this variability were examined, a number of behavioral, social, psychological, and health status variables were found to be important predictors of change in physical activity level. At age 70, men and women who smoked showed a 1.63 and 1.65-fold, respectively, greater decline in physical activity compared to never smokers, with

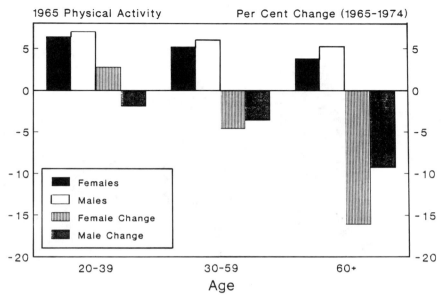

FIG. 3.5. Baseline level of leisure-time physical activity and 1965–1974
change in leisure-time physical activity by age and sex.

adjustment for body mass index and baseline level of physical activity. Body
mass index was also related to declines in physical activity; among those 60
years old or more, thin men showing especially large declines. Not surprisingly, incidence of cardiovascular conditions during the follow-up was also associated with greater declines in physical activity. Those over 70 who were socially isolated showed greater declines than those who were not isolated with
2.3-fold and 4.4-fold greater declines in isolated men and women, respectively. Men and women who were not married had approximately 30% greater
declines over 9 years, as did those with less than a high school education (1.3-fold
and 1.6-fold women and men, respectively). Depression, low life satisfaction,
and being Black versus White were also associated with greater declines at
age 70.

In a similar manner, the natural history of social isolation has also been
studied (Kaplan, Lazarus, Cohen, & Leu, 1991). Among those who were not
socially isolated in 1965, the 9-year risk of becoming socially isolated varied
by age and sex (Fig. 3.6). Men generally had higher risks, and the risk of becoming socially isolated declined with increasing age. For women, the highest
risks were among the youngest and declined until age 60, at which point they
increased. Closer inspection indicated that at age 70 and above, the risks for
women exceeded those for men. In general, the results indicate, consistent with

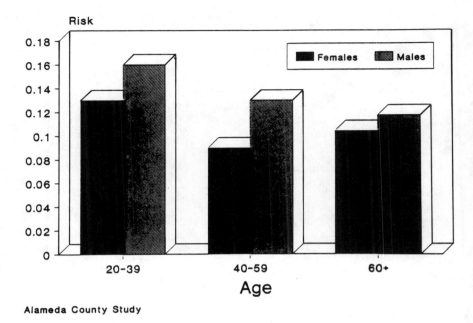

FIG. 3.6. Risk of social isolation (1965–1974) by age and sex.

other studies, that the stereotype of the elderly becoming progressively isolated is not correct. As in the case of changes in physical activity it was possible
to examine what factors were associated with increasing risk of social isolation. Again, there was a wide array of behavioral, social, psychological, health
status, and demographic factors that were related to risk of social isolation in
1965. Being disabled, or becoming disabled, were both associated with increased
risk. For example, in women, difficulties in performing ADLs in 1965 were
associated with a 2.3-fold increased risk of being socially isolated in 1974 (95%
Confidence Interval, 1.38-3.92). Low levels of physical activity were also associated with increased risk of social isolation, with a greater effect for women
than for men. Psychological factors such as depression and low life satisfaction
were also associated with increased risk of social isolation. Finally, there was
an almost linear relationship between the number of negative life events experienced between 1965-1974 and the risk of social isolation (Fig. 3.7).

OVERALL PATTERN OF RESULTS

Figure 3.8 summarizes the results seen in the analyses reported here, and in
others not reported here. A " + " indicates that a significant association has
been seen, a "0" indicates that no association was found, and a blank indicates

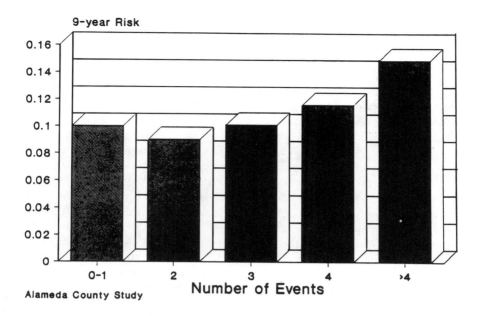

FIG. 3.7. Risk of social isolation (1965–1974) by negative life events (1965–1974) for those 60+ years.

	Death	ADL's	Physical Function	Physical Activity	Depression	Isolation
Health Status	+	+	+	+	+	+
Perceived Health	+	+	0	+	+	+
Physical Activity	+	+	+		+	+
Smoking	+	+	+	+	0	0
Relative Weight	+	+	+	0	0	
Alcohol	+	0	+	0	0	
Marital Status	0	+	+	+	0	+
Group Member	+	0	+	+	+	+
Isolation	+	+		+	+	
Social Networks	+	+		+	+	+
Race	0	+	+	+	0	+
Education	0	+	+	+	+	0
Income	0	+	+	+	0	0
Area Properties	+	+			0	
Depression	+	+	+	+		+
Life Satisfaction	+	+		+	+	+
Personal Uncer.	+	+		+	+	0
Life Events	+	+			+	+

+ = significant association   0 = not significant   blank = not studied

FIG. 3.8. Summary of predictors and outcomes for those 60+ years.

83

that the association has not been examined. As can be seen, a given variable may be related to multiple outcomes, and some variables serve as both predictors and outcomes. The predominant pattern is one of mutual determination, with little evidence of any simple causal pathways. The complexity of the results are seen even when we consider only a few outcomes and predictors (Fig. 3.9). Depression, social isolation, physical activity, and problems in performing activities of daily living, are all interconnected. Levels of depression are predictive of subsequent levels of physical activity, social isolation, or ADLs. Similarly, social isolation predicts subsequent levels of depression, physical activity, and ADLs. To complete the circle, levels of ADLs are predictive of subsequent levels of physical activity, depression, and social isolation. The impact of depression on risk of death appears to be largely through these variables and others related to health status, whereas the three other variables are independent predictors of mortality risk. Of course, the situation is much more complex when the impact of other variables is added. In fact a major need is the development of models that allow the full complexity of these relationships and their causal connections to be explicated.

It is not really surprising that the health and functioning of older persons should be affected by a wide range of variables. What remains to be more fully understood are the dynamics of this process, and the physiologic pathways that

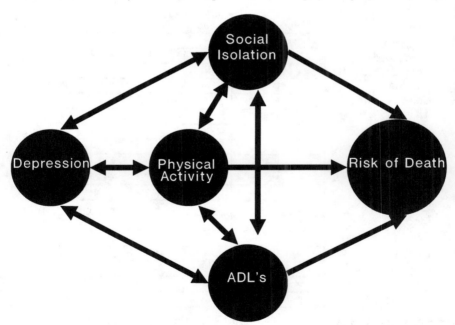

FIG. 3.9. Interrelationships between social isolation, physical activity, depression, functional health, and risk of death.

mediate these associations. It is clear that the understanding of these relationships and processes will require studies that assess a broad range of behavioral,
social, demographic, psychological, and physiologic variables—far broader,
even, than those studied in the Alameda County Study. In addition, a full understanding of the dynamic patterns of interaction between all these variables
will require studies that carry out multiple assessments over time.

THE MEANING OF AGING IN EPIDEMIOLOGIC RESEARCH

A full appreciation of the pathways by which health, in all its manifestations,
is determined for older persons, will also require some continued thinking about
the interpretation of "age" in epidemiologic research. Although it is clear that
researchers have moved away from simply dealing with age as a nuisance or
adjustment variable, there still needs to be further consideration of what age
represents and how it affects health. The importance of distinguishing age,
period, and cohort effects continues to be an important agenda, and one that
has not been adequately addressed in health-related research. Given the pau-
city of databases that would allow these factors to be properly studied, we need
to continue to keep in mind that age differences observed in a longitudinal study
may carry with them important behavioral, social, and demographic differences that are cohort-related.

It is clear that conclusions reached about the aging process from the observation of cross-sectional age differences are likely to misinform us. But even
conclusions that derive from longitudinal studies may not be without problems
in interpretation. Leaving the issues of age-period-cohort analysis aside, it is
not clear that conclusions reached from prospective studies will necessarily yield
information about the aging process, per se. The reason for this is that aging
does not take place in a vacuum. Instead, there are exposures, challenges, and
problems that occur in an age-related way. The clearest examples relate to events
such as retirement and bereavement, but there are others. Unless studies of
aging take into account these socioenvironmental events, and the behavioral,
cognitive, and psychological responses to these events, then the conclusions
about "aging" will be importantly confounded. To give a more specific example, consider possible age-dependent changes in pulmonary function and
in exercise capacity. These changes, which vary greatly from individual to individual, reflect a combination of the physiological aging of individuals, and,
perhaps to an even greater extent, represent the consequences of exposures
to various factors such as tobacco and physical exercise. Tobacco exposure and
participating in exercise are of course individual decisions, but these decisions
are greatly influenced by societal attitudes, environmental controls (tobacco)
or opportunities (exercise), and by societal expectations about what is appro-

priate at a given age. Thus, when patterns of change with age of pulmonary function and exercise capacity are studied, even longitudinally, we are looking at a process which involves far more than just aging. In the same sense that geneticists study the interaction of genotype and environment, students of aging, by necessity, must study the interaction of age and environment.

With these issues in mind, there needs to be a continued epidemiologic emphasis on a number of key questions which have not been addressed in most studies. Among these are the following:

1. Are there changes in the associations between risk factors and morbidity and mortality with increasing age? Do these changes represent selection effects; cumulative effects of exposures over a lifetime; changes in the social, behavioral, and psychological environment; or other factors?

2. Do the predictors of change in risk factors vary by age? If so, can an understanding of the ways in which environments, demands, and resources change with age advance our ability to construct efficacious interventions?

3. Can an emphasis on the behavioral, social, psychological, demographic, and environmental situations that are unique to particular ages help us to understand the development of age-dependent diseases (Brody & Schneider, 1986)?

4. Does lifetime exposure to behavioral, social, and other risk factors influence the impact of age-dependent risk factors such as bereavement?

5. Can the contribution of behavioral, social, psychological, demographic, and environmental factors to both incidence and progression of age-dependent diseases be understood? This is an issue of critical importance to the controversy concerning the compression of morbidity.

CONCLUSIONS

These results from the Alameda County Study, and other analyses, underscore the importance of a broad approach to the study of aging and health. There appears to be dense, reciprocal determination of a broad range of behavioral, social, psychological, and demographic risk factors. The proper study of systems of this complexity will require study designs and analytic techniques which strain our current resources and knowledge. From a public health perspective, however, such studies will be necessary to provide a firm basis for a new disease prevention/health promotion approach that can reduce the burden of disease, illness, and disability in an aging population.

REFERENCES

Berkman, L. F., & Breslow, L. (1983). *Health and ways of living: The Alameda County Study*. New York: Oxford University Press.

Brody, J. A., Dwight, B. B., & Williams, T. F. (1987). Trends in the health of the elderly population. *Annual Review of Public Health, 8,* 211–234.

Brody, J. A., & Schneider, E. L. (1989). Diseases and disorders of aging: A hypothesis. *Journal of Chronic Diseases, 39*(11), 871–876.

Fries, J. F. (1980). Aging, natural death, and the compression of morbidity. *New England Journal of Medicine, 303,* 130–135.

Fries, J. F. (1983). The compression of morbidity. *Milbank Memorial Fund Quarterly, 61,* 397–419.

Fries, J. F. (1984). The compression of morbidity: miscellaneous comments. *Gerontologist, 24,* 354–359.

Guralnik, J. M. (1985). *Determinants of functional health status in the elderly.* Unpublished doctoral dissertation, University of California, Berkeley, CA.

Guralnik, J. M., & Kaplan, G. A. (1989). Predictors of healthy aging: prospective evidence from the Alameda County Study. *American Journal of Public Health, 79*(6), 703–708.

Haan, M., Kaplan, G. A., & Camacho, T. (1987). Poverty and health: prospective evidence from the Alameda County Study. *American Journal of Epidemiology, 125*(6), 989–998.

Hochstim, J. R. (1970). Health and ways of living—the Alameda County, California, population laboratory. In I. I. Kessler & M. L. Levin (Eds.), *The community as an epidemiologic laboratory* (pp. 149–176). Baltimore, MD: Johns Hopkins University Press.

Kannel, W. B., & Gordon, T. (1980). Cardiovascular risk factors in the aged: The Framingham Study. In S. Haynes & M. Feinleib (Eds.), *Second conference on the epidemiology of aging.* Bethesda, MD: National Institutes of Health (No. 80-969).

Kaplan, G. A. (1985). Psychosocial aspects of chronic illness: direct and indirect associations with ischemic heart disease mortality. In R. M. Kaplan & M. H. Criqui (Eds.), *Behavioral epidemiology and disease prevention* (pp. 237–269). New York: Plenum.

Kaplan, G. A., & Camacho, T. (1983). Perceived health and mortality: Nine-year follow-up of the Human Population Laboratory cohort. *American Journal of Epidemiology, 117*(3), 292–304.

Kaplan, G. A., & Haan, M. N. (1989). Is there a role for prevention among the elderly? Epidemiologic evidence from the Alameda County Study. In M. G. Ory & K. Bond (Eds.), *Aging and health care: social science and policy perspectives* (pp. 27–51). London: Tavistock.

Kaplan, G. A., Lazarus, N. B., Cohen, R. D., & Leu, D. J. (1991). *The natural history of social isolation: Prospective evidence from the Alameda County Study.* Manuscript submitted for publication.

Kaplan, G. A., & Reynolds, P. (1988). Depression and cancer mortality and morbidity: prospective evidence from the Alameda County Study. *Journal of Behavioral Medicine, 11,* 1–13.

Kaplan, G. A., Roberts, R. E., Camacho, T. C., & Coyne, J. C. (1987). Psychosocial predictors of depression: prospective evidence from the Human Population Laboratory Studies. *American Journal of Epidemiology, 125*(2), 206–220.

Kaplan, G. A., Seeman, T. E., Cohen, R. D., Knudsen, L. P., & Guralnik, J. (1987). Mortality among the elderly in the Alameda County Study: Behavioral and demographic risk factors. *American Journal of Public Health, 77,* 307–312.

Lazarus, N. B., Kaplan, G. A., & Cohen, R. D. (1991). *Change in alcohol consumption and risk of death from all causes and from cardiovascular causes.* Manuscript submitted for publication.

Lazarus, N. B., Kaplan, G. A., Cohen, R. D., & Leu, D. J. (1989). Smoking and body mass in the natural history of physical activity: prospective evidence from the Alameda County Study, 1965–1974. *American Journal of Preventive Medicine, 5*(3), 127–135.

Manton, K. G. (1982). Changing concepts of morbidity and mortality in the elderly population. *Milbank Memorial Fund Quarterly, 60,* 183–244.

Manton, K. G., & Soldo, B. J. (1985). Dynamics of health change in the oldest old: New perspectives and evidence. *Milbank Memorial Fund Quarterly, 63,* 206–285.

National Center for Health Statistics. (1988). *Health, United States, 1987* (DHHS Pub. No. [PHS] 88-1232). Washington, DC: U.S. Government Printing Office.

Riley, M. W. (1981). Health behavior of older people: Toward a new paradigm. In D. L. Parron, F. Solomon, & J. Rodin (Eds.), *Health, behavior, and aging: a research agenda.* Washington, DC: Institute of Medicine.

Roberts, R. E., Kaplan, G. A., & Camacho, T. C. (1990). Psychological distress and mortality: Evidence from the Alameda County Study. *Social Science & Medicine, 31*(5), 527–536.

Rowe, J. W., & Kahn, R. L. (1987). Human aging: Usual and successful. *Science, 237*, 143–149.

Schneider, E. L., & Brody, J. A. (1983). Aging, natural death and the compression of morbidity: another view. *New England Journal of Medicine, 309*, 854–855.

Schneider, E. L., & Guralnik, J. M. (1987). The compression of morbidity: A dream which may come true, someday. *Gerontologica Perspecta, 1*, 8–14.

Seeman, T. E., Guralnik, J. M., Kaplan, G. A., Knudsen, L., & Cohen, R. (1989). The health consequences of multiple morbidity in the elderly: the Alameda County Study. *Journal of Aging & Health, 1*(1), 50–66.

Seeman, T. E., Kaplan, G. A., Knudsen, L., Cohen, R., & Guralnik, J. (1987). Social network ties and mortality among the elderly in the Alameda County Study. *American Journal of Epidemiology, 126*(4), 714–723.

Vaupel, J. W., & Yashin, A. I. (1985). Heterogeneity's ruses: some surprising effects of selection on population dynamics. *American Statistician, 39*, 176–185.

Wingard, D. L., Cohn, B. A., Kaplan, G. A., Cirillo, P. M., & Cohen, R. D. (1989). Sex differentials in morbidity and mortality risk examined by age and cause in the same cohort. *American Journal of Epidemiology, 130*(3), 601–610.

Aging and the Public Health: Reflections on Kaplan's Report of Health and Aging in the Alameda County Study

Ilene C. Siegler
Duke University

The Alameda County Study was designed as a prospective epidemiologic study to evaluate the role of social and psychological factors in health with a particular emphasis on cancer outcomes. Although follow-up in traditional epidemiologic studies has generally been concerned with the measurement of disease outcomes and mortality, the inclusion of repeated measures of risk factors, confounders, and effect modifiers have made traditional epidemiologic studies such as the Alameda County Study an excellent source of longitudinal information that can be used to study aging processes. Kaplan's excellent presentation provides an introduction to the possibilities inherent in the study.

Kaplan reviews his own and colleagues' contributions of the data to understanding how social, demographic, behavioral, and psychological factors influence the health status of the elderly. It is interesting to realize that the Alameda County Study is a population survey without serial medical examinations (cf. e.g., the Framingham Study, Dawber, 1980). This illustrates the contributions that can be made with survey methodology and self-reports of conditions, symptoms, and archival data available about the Alameda County community added to the information available from death certificates. The implications of data from such studies has been recently discussed with intelligence and insight by Elias, Elias, and Elias (1990) in their chapter for the third revision of the *Handbook of Psychology of Aging*. They pointed out that there are limitations without medical confirmation of the types of conclusions that can be drawn from health surveys as well as provide an excellent review of current age-based thinking about health and behavior.

In this discussion, I first use Kaplan's chapter as a springboard for a discussion of four themes suggested by his work and second, I give one set of answers to the questions he ended with. The four themes to be discussed are:

1. Aging and the public health. This has implications of enhanced survival, and the meaning of prevention (of mortality?) as a goal in the epidemiology of aging, and the inclusion of non-mortality outcomes such as functional health and risk factor change;
2. The meaning of age as an adjustment variable in classical epidemiologic models;
3. The meaning of time in an epidemiology of aging: What is on time for disease? Are there different risk factors for premature disease versus on-time disease versus later disease? and
4. Possible models of research design that will blend the best of life-span developmental psychology with epidemiology.

REFLECTIONS ON HEALTH AND AGING

Aging and the Public Health

Concern with understanding the implications of an aging society (Neugarten & Neugarten, 1989) for research and practice in public health is relatively recent (Phillips & Gaylord, 1985), and not surprising, given the aging of many epidemiologic study cohorts. However, traditional public health concepts and methods have generally treated age as variance to be controlled for, rather than explained.

Implications of Enhanced Survival. First, someone must be doing a good job with enhanced survival. If long life is a goal of public health then more and more U.S. citizens are achieving it (if they make it out of the high risk periods of infancy and adolescence). Once adulthood is achieved, then long life is becoming normative. In 1985, 70% of the U.S. population survived to the age of 65 and 30% survived until at least 80 years of age (Brody, Brock, & Williams, 1987). Kaplan is correct in stating that the elderly differ today. One of the most important ways is in their age, they are older; and in the expectation that they will live to become aged. Given the Alameda County Study started with a population aged 16–94, they have the capacity to observe multiple generations of the elderly. Verbrugge (1989) discussed the implications of changes in mortality in the context of population morbidity or "longer life but worsening health" (p. 333). Although her discussion of the issues was excellent, what is surprising, is how little actual data we have on individuals to test such notions. This is being remedied.

Public Health is Primarily Concerned With Prevention. This preoccupation does not translate into aging. Can we really prevent mortality? Aside from the science fiction aspects of such a question, we have succeeded in getting a fair share of morbidity into the later years such that 60 does not seem old any more. Prevention of disability and prevention of frailty now make sense as research questions and as policy goals. However, we do not generally study or have models of the risk of the burden of illness in developmental psychology. There are models in public health (German & Fried, 1989), and the analyses presented by Kaplan represent an important contribution to this research effort (see Tables 3.1 and 3.2).

What is the Meaning of All-Cause Mortality as an Outcome?   The outcome in all-cause mortality is length of life. This implies that quantity not quality of life is important (Siegler, 1990). We rarely, on our studies, follow persons to determine the point at which there is a drop in the quality of life that is a meaningful date to put into an analysis. It would, however, be an interesting measurement strategy to design. Because ascertainment of date of death can be accomplished through sources such as the National Death Index or State Vital Statistics Offices, it is a "relatively" simple endpoint to measure.

Aside from what quantity of life means, as I have argued elsewhere (Siegler, 1989), this choice of survival as a dependent variable is a consequential decision if one wishes to have a health psychology (Rodin & Salovey, 1989) that includes a knowledge about how age works in conjunction with health. I think that cause-specific mortality tells us more about the particular mechanisms of a disease. Matthews (1989), in her Presidential Address to Division 38, made a wonderful case for the specificity gained in studies of coronary disease; as did the examples she gave in her discussion at this conference.

Age as an Adjustment Variable

Kaplan's chapter is a decided improvement from the traditional epidemiologic approach of only reporting effects that remain after controlling for age because he only controlled for age *within* the elderly age range. However, it may be that between the ages of 70 and 94 questions about how age operates at 70 versus how it operates at 94 would be instructive. But one is tempted to ask why the results are reported for only particular segments of the age population and not the full range of ages; and why the summary of factors such as found in Fig. 3.8, is not at least given for the younger half of the Alameda County sample so that over the same 19-year observation period, one could compare and contrast the evidence of the risk factors and outcomes for those initially aged under 70 as well as those aged 70 and older. Kaplan's chapter makes me greedy for more findings. I want another Fig. 3.8 with all of the findings summarized for members of the Alameda County Study population aged 30–59. His text gives some clues as to what such a figure would look like. Risk factors that appear to predict survival (net of covariates) for those under the age of

70 but not for those 70 and older are: being unmarried, being Black, having lower levels of education and income, being depressed, and, furthermore that the older group is less likely to have an increase in social isolation. It is interesting that these are primarily sociodemographic factors that determine who gets selected into the elderly; but once selected, different factors may come into play. It would be extremely instructive to know; and leads to my next question:

The Meanings of Time

What is On-Time Disease?   It is important to ask what it means to have an age-dependent disease; and what it means when that disease is moved later on in the life cycle perhaps due to changes in risk factors—or moved earlier in the life cycle due to scientific advances that lead to detection in asymptomatic phases of the disease. This can be expected to vary by disease and to change over time.

Kaplan finds that the traditional behavioral risk factors predict 17-year mortality within the elderly aged 70–94 at about the same rate (see Fig. 3.2). Adjusted for age, gender, and baseline health, smoking adds 43%, inactivity 37%, heavy drinking 39%, and extremes of relative weight 32%. This contradicts the conventional wisdom that risk factors no longer matter in later life. Kuller (1989), in an editorial accompanying an article from the Honolulu Heart Study by Benfante, Reed, Mac Lean and Yano (1989), pointed up the fact that there are a lot of unanswered questions. The Alameda County Study can help provide the answers. The results of Benfante et al. (1989) argue that special attention to age at onset of a disease and strength of risk factors within different age groups will be a productive avenue of study. In addition, they present some modifications to traditional epidemiologic methods needed to calculate the period of risk for each subject.

Model Research Designs

Kaplan's chapter was noteworthy in attempting to model a proxy for the aging process by looking at incident health problems predicting incident ADL problems (Table 3.2). It might also be instructive to use prospective database to predict change in the outcomes (e.g., stable IQ vs. declining IQ) and to put change patterns predicting change outcomes as in using difference scores in canonical analyses. That might better capture some of the truth of what is really happening in the aging process. Schaie (1989), in his Kleemeier Award lecture, proposed the application of life-history analyses to problems in the psychology of adult development and aging (see Schaie, 1989, pp. 487–489 for a cogent explanation). Such methodological modeling will become increasingly important. In discussing the meaning of aging in epidemiologic research, Kaplan states, "it is not clear that conclusions reached from prospective studies will necessarily yield information about the aging process, per se." This is true now; but need not stay that way. Some design modifications will be required. In particular, collection of more than just mortality and single disease outcome data after baseline is helpful as the collection of later risk factor data in the Alameda County Study illustrated. Second, following all members of the cohort, not just those "disease free" for outcomes aside from mortality will increase our knowledge of the natural history of diseases and of aging with a disease. Third, finding sets of intermediate outcomes that serve as markers of aging—successful and unsuccessful aging if those can be defined is a critical challenge for the future.

Older persons are influenced by "popular culture" as are younger persons—particularly the well-educated and moderately well-off. Thus, risk factor changes happening in the elderly can be expected to be the norm. We need models that deal with changes in risk behaviors as well as in outcomes that change in their likelihood after a specific age. The presentation by Kaplan was an excellent step in this direction.

A SET OF ANSWERS

Dr. Kaplan ended his talk with a series of questions by way of summarizing his main points. I provide one set of answers:

1. In answer to the questions about changes in associations between risk factors and morbidity and mortality—yes! I think his possible explanations for any observed associations are likely candidates that should be formally evaluated (e.g., selection, cumulative exposures, changes in environments) and that this important question implies more important questions to be asked: When does morbidity become a risk for mortality and does it differ as a function of age at onset? Are there specific ages of onset that once passed make the risk for a disorder or cause of death decrease with age?

2. Do predictors of change in risk factors vary by age? My best guess would be no. My assumption is that changes in risk factor behaviors are mediated by time of measurement effects and that at any given time, economic and social status, rather than age, control the variation of who has the luxury to modify a risk factor.

3. I do not know what it means to have behavioral, social, psychological, demographic, and environmental situations unique to particular ages. In general, situations—such as wars (see Siegler & George, 1983) happen to families and impact unevenly across the birth cohorts. Society does not appear to be age stratified in a linear fashion, as this question suggests. Birren (1959) in the first *Handbook of Aging and the Individual* discussed the meaning of age as an explanatory variable:

> Chronological age is a powerful index with which we can classify large amounts of data while seeking relationships. Unless we can attach some significance to

the role of time or age in the large array of facts in which it is imbedded, we might argue that the value of chronological age is limited to that of a pervasive filing index for data we cannot otherwise classify. (p. 8)

There are many interesting questions about age-dependent diseases that I would like to know that may really be a restatement of Kaplan's original question. What makes a disease appear early, on time, or late? Or to use Benfante et al.'s cut point over or under the age of 60 for coronary heart disease.

4. Why is bereavement an age-dependent risk factor? It is my understanding that coping with the death of a loved one is much more difficult when the death is that of a child and widowhood is more stressful for those where it is least expected.

5. The answer is definitely yes, non-medical factors have a major contribution to make to our understanding of the compression of morbidity, although as Verbrugge (1989) pointed out, there is no evidence that there is a compression of morbidity as yet.

A FINAL COMMENT

A major emergent issue for me that has been stimulated by this chapter is the question of what is the proper outcome for health/behavior/aging research. I think the prediction of length of survival is less interesting once we are no longer talking about premature mortality. Rather that we should be predicting the onset of frailty, the timing of disability, the onset of diseases that have their appearance in later life, or, in a sense, the disappearance of health. This disappearance of health may become a new operational definition for aging.

ACKNOWLEDGMENTS

Dr. Siegler's work is supported by Grant P01-HL36587 from National Heart Lung and Blood Institute and Grant P50-AG05128 from the National Institute on Aging. I would like to thank Harry T. Phillips, MD, DPH who started me thinking about the intersection of aging and public health.

REFERENCES

Benfante, R. J., Reed, D. M., Mac Lean, C. J., & Yano, K. (1989). Risk factors in middle age that predict early and late onset of coronary heart disease. *Journal of Clinical Epidemiology, 42*(2), 95–104.

Birren, J. E. (1959). Principles of research on aging. In J. E. Birren (Ed.), *Handbook of aging and the individual: Psychological and biological aspects* (pp. 3–42). Chicago: University of Chicago Press.

Brody, J. A., Brock, D. B., & Williams, T. F. (1987). Trends in the health of the elderly population. In L. Breslow, J. E. Fielding, & L. B. Lave (Eds.), *Annual review of public health* (Vol. 8, pp. 211–234). Palo Alto: Annual Reviews.

Dawber, T. R. (1980). *The Framingham Study: The epidemiology of atherosclerotic disease*. Cambridge MA: Harvard University Press.

Elias, M. F., Elias, J. K., & Elias, P. K. (1990). Biological and health influences on behavior. In J. E. Birren & K. W. Schaie (Eds.), *Handbook of the psychology of aging* (3rd ed., pp. 79–102). New York: Academic Press.

German, P. S., & Fried, L. P. (1989). Prevention and the elderly: Public health issues and strategies. *Annual review of public health* (Vol. 10, pp. 319–32). Palo Alto: Annual Reviews.

Matthews, K. A. (1989). Interactive effects of behavior and reproductive hormones on sex differences in risk for coronary disease. *Health Psychology, 8*(4), 373–388.

Neugarten, B. L. & Neugarten, D. A. (1989). Policy issues in an aging society. In M. Storandt & G. R. VandenBos (Eds.), *The adult years: Continuity and change* (pp. 147–167). Washington, DC: American Psychological Association.

Phillips, H. T., & Gaylord, S. A. (Eds.). (1985). *Aging and public health*. New York: Springer.

Rodin, J., & Salovey, P. (1989). Health psychology. In M. R. Rosenzweig & L. W. Porter (Eds.), *Annual review of psychology* (Vol. 40, pp. 533–79). Palo Alto: Annual Reviews.

Schaie, K. W. (1989). The hazards of cognitive aging. *The Gerontologist, 29*(4), 484–493.

Siegler, I. C. (1989). Developmental health psychology. In M. Storandt & G. R. VandenBos (Eds.), *The adult years: Continuity and change* (pp. 119–142). Washington, DC: American Psychological Association.

Siegler, I. C. (1990). Intelligence, personality and longevity. In R. T. Mc Carter & D. Park (Co-chairs), *Aging processes: Phylogenetic and cognitive approaches*. American Association for the Advancement of Science Meetings, New Orleans, LA.

Siegler, I. C., & George, L. K. (1983). Sex differences in coping and perceptions of life events. *Journal of Geriatric Psychiatry, 16*(2), 197–209.

Verbrugge, L. M. (1989). Recent, present and future health of American adults. *Annual Review of Public Health, 10*, 333–61.

The Laudables and Limits of Large Epidemiologic Studies of Mortality

Dan Blazer
Duke University Medical Center

The Alameda County Study is a prototype of community-based morbidity and mortality studies. The investigative team, of which Dr. Kaplan has been an integral member and now director, has utilized this cohort and existing data banks as extensively and productively as any group of investigators in the United States. In his chapter, Dr. Kaplan has reviewed for us in great detail the variety of risk factors for morbidity and mortality available for study, and has informed us where positive associations have been found, where no associations have been found, and what areas remain for future study. He has also reviewed a series of questions that provide a next step of analyses that, I am certain, he will pursue with great diligence.

Let me return, however, to the "so what?" questions that I posed as goals for this volume. I am the only physician among the participants. Therefore, I ignore my social epidemiology background for a few minutes and address the findings of the Alameda County Study regarding one risk factor—alcohol use, as a physician treating older adults who use alcohol on a regular basis. I recognize that these comments appear provocative and even unsophisticated. They are delivered, however, in the service of sharpening the focus of the participants upon the meaning of their past investigative efforts and directions for the future investigations. If these comments stimulate challenges and rebuttals, they will have served their purpose.

I related the four questions that I asked previously to alcohol use in the elderly as a risk factor. First, "so what" is the true nature and characteristic of this risk factor labeled "alcohol use" (and defined as 45 or more drinks per month). The patterns of alcohol use that I observe in my practice are many and the quantity of alcohol use over a given month appears uninformative regarding both short- and long-term morbidity and mortality. I describe four such patterns.

The first pattern is the "skid row" alcoholic who may drink as much as a pint of alcohol a day (or even more). His or her alcohol intake is clearly much greater than 45 drinks a month and the adverse effects on his or her health are multiple. His or her life expectancy is limited and functioning is impaired directly by continual alcohol use, not to mention the chronic physical problems suffered through continued excessive use of alcohol. He or she may suffer many injuries secondary to drinking (e.g., fractures, burns) as well as chronic deterioration of health. A second pattern of an older adult suffering a problem with alcohol is "two martini lunch and wine for dinner for 50 years." These patients seek consultation (usually at the encouragement of the family) because of a decline in their functional capabilities during their 60s or 70s. Memory loss is the most common presenting symptom. Many of these elders who suffer difficulties with memory have actually decreased their alcohol intake to one drink a day with occasional drinks at other times (i.e., no longer drinking 45 drinks a month). Nevertheless, every ounce of alcohol increases the risk for increased impairment in this older adult who, through many years of exposure, is especially sensitive to the toxic effects of alcohol.

The third pattern I encounter is the "binge drinker." This older adult may actually begin drinking late in life, possibly after a move to a retirement community. He or she may be suffering difficulties with adjustment and these difficulties may have precipitated a depressive disorder, which is the reason this person has resorted to alcohol. Counting drinks per month does not assist us in understanding the problem the person suffers with alcohol. This older adult may binge two or three times per month drinking 10 drinks during a "binge." During a binge, he or she may become acutely suicidal, suffer blackouts, fall, and fail to perform many regular daily activities. Risks from morbidity and mortality are great during a binge but during the alcohol free periods, this person actually functions at a normal level.

The fourth pattern that I encounter, the "colleague," that is, the person we may encounter socially who drinks two drinks per day every day of the year. He or she suffers no problems with intoxication, his or her memory is intact, and every laboratory test performed to determine if this person suffers toxic physical effects from the alcohol is negative. Does he or she have a problem with alcohol? Should I be concerned about his or her alcohol intake? On occasions, the risk factors used by epidemiologists appear sterile within the context of the patterns of alcohol use I encounter as a clinician.

"So what" are the mechanisms by which social factors impact disease onset, disease outcomes, health maintenance, and enhancement? Identifying a risk factor for morbidity and mortality, such as the use of alcohol, should encourage theories of the mechanisms by which alcohol might increase the risk for a poor outcome. Clinical observations should contribute to epidemiologic studies in the future. For example, poor nutritional status, neglect of health during the midst of alcohol use, social isolation related to alcohol use, the use of alcohol to cover psychiatric disorders that may lead the elder to an increased risk of morbidity and mortality (such as depressive disorders) and falls are possible mechanisms, in addition to the direct physical effects of alcohol such as cirrhosis and dementia. The relative contribution of each of these potential adverse effects of alcohol use/abuse can be explored through community and clinical based epidemiologic inquiry.

"So what" are the public health implications of the findings that alcohol use leads to an increased risk for morbidity and mortality? To place the question in a more practical perspective, should the clinician treating a healthy and mentally alert older adult initiate vigorous intervention plans to reduce alcohol use in patients who seek consultation for other reasons. Physicians often do encourage such changes in health behavior, especially in the area of smoking cessation, even if the presenting problem to the clinician is totally unrelated. Although epidemiologic studies per se do not provide a specific "take home" message for clinicians regarding the need to encourage reduction or cessation of alcohol use, these studies can inform clinicians regarding the relative risk of continued alcohol use, especially when data are presented suggesting that alcohol use can be a significant risk factor when associated with other risk factors. For example, alcohol use does become a public health issue for clinicians when it is associated with social isolation, a decline in physical health, impulsive behavior, and significant symptoms of depression. The addictive and interactive effects of alcohol with other risk factors are important determinants of the risk for suicide, not an infrequent public health problem among older adults.

"So what" are the next studies that will advance our understanding of disease onset, disease progression, prevention of disease, functional impairment, and mortality? Should we continue large-scale studies? Should we emphasize supplemental studies to ongoing large-scaled studies such as the NHANES or the EPESEs? Should we proceed with more intensive studies of smaller numbers of subjects? Should clues for epidemiologic community studies be transferred to the laboratory for further inquiry? Have we enough data to field large scale intervention studies, such as the Mr. Fit studies to prevent cardiovascular disease? The answer to this question, in the area of alcohol abuse/dependence is "all of the above." Epidemiology clearly can inform clinicians and the general public regarding the nature and extent of alcohol problems among older adults. Epidemiologic studies also inform the scientific community at large regarding the nature of the association between alcohol use and a variety of health outcome measures. These studies are first steps toward a variety of additional studies that span clinical medicine and psychiatry.

If these epidemiologic studies are to be of value, they must be meaningful to both the laboratory scientists studying the mechanisms of changes that take place in the body and the brain of the older adult using alcohol and the clinician who treats the older adult who drinks alcohol regularly and/or who suffers from alcohol related problems. Meaning, however, does not imply relevance. Science cannot move forward if it feels constrained that every scientific endeavor must be ''relevant'' to clinical practice. Nevertheless, clinicians can inform the social scientist and the epidemiologist so that epidemiologic inquiries are not sterile but rather are conceived and implemented within the context of the ''real world'' of the older adult exposed to a putative risk factor within a biological and social environment that interacts in many ways with that risk factor.

Dr. Kaplan's chapter provides an excellent ''first step'' in identifying a variety of risk factors and his work already has begun to explore the interaction and association of those risk factors and a variety of outcomes of importance, especially mortality and function. The context of future studies that derive from the findings by Dr. Kaplan and his colleagues will become increasingly important, however.

If context is a focus of these studies, then they will prove meaningful to the interdisciplinary community studying these problems.

Living Arrangements and Problems With Daily Tasks for Older Women With Breast Cancer

William A. Satariano
University of California

Nawal E. Ragheb
Michigan State University

INTRODUCTION

Breast cancer is the leading form of cancer diagnosed in women (Sondik, Young, Horm, & Ries, 1988). Once diagnosed, however, women with breast cancer have substantially better relative survival rates than those diagnosed with other leading forms of cancer, such as colon cancer and cancers of the lung and bronchus (Sondik et al., 1987; Ries, Pollack, & Young, 1983). The large number of breast cancer cases diagnosed each year, plus the relatively favorable survival rates for treated patients, suggest that the quality of that survival is an important issue.

Quality of survival has been assessed in a variety of ways. In most cases, research has been devoted to psychosocial aspects of adjustment (Taylor et al., 1985; Thomas, 1978). Less attention has been paid to more general areas of functioning, such as the degree of difficulty in completing physical tasks and the ease with which instrumental activities of daily living can be completed.

Instrumental activities of daily living (IADL), especially those dealing with tasks necessary to maintain independence in the home (housekeeping, grocery shopping and meal preparation) deserve special attention. IADL functioning is generally regarded as one of the standard methods of assessing the need for long-term care services (Kane & Kane, 1987; Kavesh, 1986; Lawton, 1972). Those people who either cannot complete these activities themselves or have the activities completed for them are more likely to be subsequently institutionalized than are those who can meet these needs for themselves (Branch, 1984; Branch & Jette, 1982). Each of the three instrumental activities corresponds directly to a specific type of home-care service. Thus, the measurement of IADL provides a means of identifying the types of services that might be needed.

Our own research in this area suggests that the satisfactory completion of IADL activities is especially problematic within the first 3 months following diagnosis of breast cancer among women aged 55 to 84 (Satariano, Ragheb, Buck, Swanson, & Branch, 1989). Regardless of age, only 25% of the cases were able to complete all IADL tasks independently. (In this study, getting to places outside of walking distance was assessed in addition to housekeeping, grocery shopping, and meal preparation.) This level of independence was in marked contrast to that exhibited by women of the same age without the disease. Among the controls, 53%, 48%, and 30% in the youngest, middle, and oldest age groups, respectively, were able to complete all tasks. Housekeeping was especially problematic. After 1 year, most women with breast cancer, with the notable exception of those aged 65 to 74, regained normal functioning.

In light of these findings, it is important to investigate why some breast cancer patients function well, whereas others do not. Theoretically, the satisfactory completion of IADL tasks should depend on both one's physical capabilities, as affected by the stage of the breast cancer at diagnosis and the presence of comorbid health problems, as well as the number and type of available social resources.

Regarding the possible effects of social resources, a number of studies have examined the influence of social support and coping processes on the mental health of older women with breast cancer (Bloom, Ross, & Burnell, 1978; DiMatteo & Hays, 1981; Wortman & Conway, 1985). It is generally reported that social support predicts a woman's adjustment to breast cancer and contributes to her enhanced self-esteem and feelings of self-efficacy. Among married women with breast cancer, the husband's response and reactions to the disease are shown to have particular significance for successful adaptation. In a recent population-based study, a variety of measures of social support, defined to include emotional, appraisal, informational, and instrumental support, had a positive and statistically significant effect on measures of quality of life, self-esteem, and role and emotional functioning, adjusting for the effects of stage of disease and other measures of physical functioning (Vinokur, Threatt, Vinokur-Kaplan, & Satariano, 1990). Although these studies suggest that social support accounts, in part, for differences in the quality of survival following diagnosis and treatment of breast cancer, we know little about how specific social relations affect the satisfactory completion of everyday tasks, such as IADL, that are necessary for independent living.

A recent report issued by the National Research Council on the Aging Population in the Twenty-First Century identified marital status and living arrangements as among the most important social relations affecting the welfare of the elderly (Gilford, 1988). Although there is a growing body of research on the health effects of marital status and living arrangements, little is known about the extent to which these social relations affect the satisfactory completion of IADL tasks among older people with an incident chronic condition, such as breast cancer.

Unmarried women, especially those who are separated and divorced, are generally more likely than married women to be at elevated risk for poor health (Ortmeyer, 1974; Verbrugge, 1979). Unmarried women are at greater risk not only for developing specific diseases, but also for poorer survival. One's marital status may be associated with specific practices that affect the risk for health problems (Berkman, 1985). In addition, unmarried women may have less access to specific forms of social support necessary to cope with that condition. Although marriage seems to confer a healthful advantage, other studies suggest that under some circumstances married women, required to care for an ill spouse, are, in fact, "hidden patients" (Fengler & Goodrich, 1979). There is considerable evidence that the strain of caregiving may have negative effects on the psychological and physical well-being of the caring spouse (e.g., Horowitz, 1985; Moritz, Kasl, & Berkman, 1989; Zarit, Todd, & Zarit, 1986). This may be especially problematic for women who must deal with their own chronic health condition and reduced physical functioning. We know very little about women in this type of situation. Research is needed to specify the conditions of cancer care that present particular problems for elderly cancer patients who are responsible for the care of other elderly persons (Kane, 1983). An ill spouse may represent both an added burden as well as a lost or impaired source of support. As such, an ill husband may elevate the risk of difficulty in completing everyday tasks for a woman newly diagnosed and treated for invasive breast cancer.

Living arrangements and, in particular, older people who live alone, also have attracted attention in studies of elderly populations. The number of elderly women living alone has doubled in the last 15 years, with projections of a continuing increase to 1995 in the proportion of households with an elderly female living alone or with nonrelatives (Siegel & Davidson, 1984). The National Research Council (NRC) panel on research on the elderly reports that this trend toward living alone has important implications for housing needs and the demand for institutional care (Gilford, 1988). Moreover, with a decline in the proportion of the elderly living with relatives likely to continue, the NRC panel foresees an increase in the need for community social support and health services. The Commonwealth Fund also has initiated a major research effort to understand more clearly the social, economic, and health implications of living alone among the elderly (The Commonwealth Fund Commission on Elderly People Living Alone, 1987).

Investigating the impact of living alone on older women with breast cancer is important for several reasons. First, of the 8.8 million elderly people who lived alone in the United States in 1987, 80% were women. Second, living arrangements relate directly to marital status; 66% of all elderly persons living alone are widowed. Research in this area may provide some understanding of the extent to which the effects of marriage on health and functioning are due to living arrangements. (See Cafferata, 1987 for a discussion of the independent and joint effects of marriage and living arrangements.) Finally, The Commonwealth Fund reports that 1.7 million older people living alone are poor, including approximately 1.1 million elderly widows. There is also a very large group of "near-poor," defined as those with incomes below 150% of the poverty line. Together, there were more than 2.6 million widows in 1987 with incomes below $156 per week classified as poor or near-poor. This group is considered to be especially vulnerable to out-of-pocket medical costs and other unexpected expenses.

There is some evidence to suggest that people who live alone are generally in better health than those living with a person other than a spouse (Magaziner, Cadigan, Hebel, & Parry, 1988; Rubinstein, 1984). Magaziner and colleagues argued that when the health of older persons declines to the point where they can no longer carry on independently, they either move in with others, or enter a nursing home. Despite the healthy profile of those living alone, Rubinstein pointed out that approximately 25% of older people who live alone are functionally limited and 10% are unable to carry out any major daily activity. He argued that this group deserves special attention. In most cases, living alone may not be problematic for those in reasonable health. However, when an emergency strikes, people who live alone may be vulnerable to the extent they have limited access to a network of friends and relatives. People who live alone are more likely than others to use health services, primarily because informal supports are not as readily available (Cafferata, 1987).

These studies suggest that social relations and, in particular, the resources derived from those relations, may help to explain why some older women with breast cancer recuperate more satisfactorily than others. It is unknown, however, whether the living arrangements of these women affect their subsequent adjustment and, specifically, their ease in completing IADL tasks.

Our purpose is threefold. First, we determine whether the risk of problems in completing specific IADL tasks for women with incident breast cancer is greater for those who live alone, compared to those living with either a spouse or with others. Second, we consider alternative approaches for investigating living arrangements by taking into account the husband's health. Does living with an ill spouse have an adverse effect on the satisfactory completion of IADL tasks, compared to problems reported by married women with a healthy spouse? It is important to note that it is not possible, at least at this stage, to determine to what extent an ill spouse represents a psychosocial or economic burden or whether an ill spouse represents a lost source of social support. However, because data on marriage and living arrangements are presently available in medical records (or at least could be obtained with minimal effort), they represent sources of information that can be used, together with demographic and clinical data, to better predict subsequent risk of difficulty in completing IADL tasks. As such, this information may be useful in developing better discharge planning procedures. The Metropolitan Detroit Cancer Surveillance System (MDCSS) and epidemiologic surveys associated with this registry provide an opportunity to address these issues relevant to living arrangements and problems with daily tasks for older women with breast cancer.

METHODS

This study is based on data obtained for a case-control examination of the epidemiology of functional disability in older women with breast cancer. Cases were interviewed 3 months after diagnosis and again 9 months later. Population-based controls also were interviewed twice over the same period.

Case Ascertainment

All female residents of the Detroit metropolitan area aged 55 to 84, newly diagnosed with microscopically confirmed, invasive breast cancer between September 1, 1984 and March 31, 1985 were identified through the MDCSS in the Division of Epidemiology at the Michigan Cancer Foundation. The MDCSS, a participant in the Surveillance, Epidemiology, and End Results (SEER) program of the National Cancer Institute, is a population-based cancer surveillance system which encompasses the Detroit metropolitan area with 4 million residents. Medical and demographic information for all cancer cases, with the exception of non-melanoma skin cancer, is obtained from the 66 tri-county hospitals, 8 private laboratories, 15 radiation therapy clinics, and other facilities, such as hospices. In addition, casefinding and abstracting are conducted in 4 out-of-area hospitals, which also provide treatment for cancer patients from the Detroit metropolitan area. Casefinding and abstracting are performed by the Division of Epidemiology staff of 26 abstractors, through review of medical and pathology records of all facilities. As a measure of the completeness of case identification, only 1.2% of all cancer cases diagnosed among metropolitan residents are obtained through death certificates (Young, Percy, & Asire, 1981).

Case ascertainment for this study used the established MDCSS rapid reporting system, which identifies cases within 2 to 4 weeks of diagnosis. This system facilitates access to cases for earlier interview, in this case, within 2 to 4 months after diagnosis.

Cases ascertained through rapid reporting were matched to MDCSS files to determine whether any had a history of breast cancer. Women with a previous

diagnosis of breast cancer were excluded from the study, whereas those diagnosed with other forms of cancer were not. Women reporting a previous breast
cancer during the interview also were excluded as ineligible. Given that the
purpose of the study is to investigate functional status among women in a noninstitutionalized setting, cases living in long-term care facilities were not eligible. Because we feel that cases were best able to judge their health and functional status, no proxy interviews were taken.

Control Ascertainment

Female residents of the Detroit metropolitan area aged 55 to 84 were identified for enrollment into the study through telephone random-digit dialing conducted between July 1, 1984 and September 30, 1984. All three-digit telephone
prefixes for the Detroit metropolitan area were stratified by geographic area
(Wayne, Oakland, and Macomb counties) to ensure proportional representation in the population sample. A sample of number prefixes, stratified by county,
was selected. Four-digit suffixes were obtained through a computer-based random numbers generator. The number and timing of telephone dialing were
designed to ensure that each potential respondent had an opportunity to be
contacted. There were 3,511 private residences reached by telephone. Of this
number, 2,773 (78.9%) respondents agreed to provide a household census,
including age, race, name, and address of women meeting the study selection
criteria.

The number and proportion of prospective controls aged 55 to 64, 65 to
74, and 75 to 84 were based on the expected number of cases diagnosed in
those age groups over an average 7-month period in the Detroit area. These
estimates were based on data previously collected on invasive breast cancer
cases through the MDCSS.

As was done with eligible cases, prospective controls were checked against
the files maintained by the MDCSS to ensure that the women did not have
a previous or current diagnosis of breast cancer. Women presumed eligible
for inclusion as controls were sent letters explaining the purpose of the study,
and later were telephoned to arrange an appointment for an interview. The
questionnaires of women who reported a previous breast cancer during the interview were eliminated from the study as ineligible.

Interview

Of the 612 women diagnosed with breast cancer over the 7-month period, 571
(93.3%) were identified within 3 months of their diagnosis date, making them
eligible for inclusion in the study. Of the 571 eligible cases, 463 (81.1%) were

successfully interviewed between 2 and 4 months after diagnosis. By interviewing cases approximately 3 months after diagnosis, we believed they would have sufficient time at home following their initial diagnosis and treatment to adequately evaluate their functional status. There was no significant difference between interviewed and noninterviewed cases by age (x^2 = 0.23, p = 0.89), race (x^2 = 3.9, p = 0.14), or stage of disease at diagnosis (x^2 = 0.43, p = 0.93). Of the 463 cases completing the first interview, 444 were still alive and not institutionalized in a long-term care facility 9 months later. During the time between the first and second phases, 14 cases died and 5 were institutionalized. Of the 444 survivors, 422 (95.1%) were interviewed 8 to 10 months after the first interview.

Of the 647 controls selected through random-digit dialing, 539 (83.3%) completed the first interview. Interviewed and noninterviewed controls did not differ significantly by age (x^2 = 3.1, p = 0.22) or race (x^2 = 0.59, p = 0.75). Of the 539 controls interviewed in the first phase, 526 were alive and not institutionalized 9 months later. Between the first and second interview, 10 controls died and 3 were institutionalized. There were 478 (90.9%) who were successfully re-interviewed 8 to 10 months after their initial interview.

Cases and controls were first interviewed between November 1, 1984 and July 31, 1985. The second interviews were conducted between July 1, 1985 and May 30, 1986. Both interviews, requiring 45 to 60 minutes to complete, covered a variety of topic areas, including general health status, health practices, social networks and social support, physical and instrumental functioning, as well as socioeconomic status and demographic characteristics.

In this chapter, we focus only on the risks of IADL problems reported at 3 months after diagnosis. As noted previously, most difficulty is experienced at this time (Satariano, Ragheb, Buck et al., 1989). It also seems appropriate to examine the associations of IADL difficulty with living arrangements at baseline, before examining longitudinal effects.

Instrumental Activities of Daily Living

A scale, adapted from the Massachusetts Health Care Panel Study and the Framingham Disability Study, was employed to characterize the respondent's level of functioning in each of three instrumental areas (housekeeping, meal preparation, and grocery shopping) (Branch, 1988; Branch & Jette, 1981). The adapted scale was based on responses to questions dealing with whether the activity was completed as often as necessary during the past month and at what level of difficulty. A problem in the completion of an IADL task was defined in terms of whether the task was not done as often as necessary and/or was completed with difficulty. Reports of who performs the task were classified separately and tested as a covariate in the analysis.

Marital Status and Living Arrangements

Respondents were asked the number of people living in their households as well as their ages and relationships to the respondent. Following other research in this area (e.g., Magaziner et al., 1988), three categories of living arrangements were used in the final analysis: "Lives alone," "Lives with spouse," "Lives with others." "Lives with spouse" includes those respondents who either live only with their spouse or with their spouse and others.

Husband's Health

Information about the husband's health was based on the respondent's assessments of her spouse's general health. In particular, an ill spouse was defined as one who met at least one of the following criteria: (a) his health was reported as worse than other men his age; (b) he had been seriously ill in the past 12 months requiring hospitalization; (c) he required assistance in completing one or more daily activities. Information about the husband's health was later used to expand the categories of living arrangements by distinguishing between respondents with a healthy spouse and those with an ill spouse.

Covariates

We estimated the independent effects of living arrangements on each of the three IADL outcomes, adjusting for a variety of demographic, social, clinical, and functional covariates. In all, seven sets of covariates were examined for each of the three outcomes. The first set of variables included demographic and social factors: race, age, education, and reported financial adequacy to meet daily needs. Clinical variables, including stage of the breast cancer at diagnosis, radiation, and type of surgery constituted the second set. The third set included measures of reported difficulty in completing a variety of physical tasks. These measures were summarized to reflect degree of disability in four areas. The final four variables reflected degree of difficulty in upper body strength, lower body strength, balance, and fine dexterity. Our previous research showed that women with breast cancer were most likely to experience difficulty in tasks involving upper body strength (Satariano, Ragheb, Branch, & Swanson, 1990). Reports of limiting concurrent health conditions were included in the fourth set of variables: limiting heart disease, limiting hypertension, limiting arthritis, and the number of remaining diagnosed conditions. Prevalent concurrent health conditions have been shown in previous analyses to be associated with both the quality and duration of survival among members of this cohort (Satariano, Ragheb, & DuPuis, 1989). Outside social con-

acts represented the fifth set: the number of personal contacts made with friends and relatives in the preceding month (Seeman, Kaplan, Knudsen, Cohen, & Guralnik, 1987). The sixth set captured other health variables including vision and auditory acuity as well as a measure of body mass. Finally, the seventh set of variables included summary measures of reported depression and fatigue.

Statistical Analyses

Logistic regression analysis was used for estimating the effects of living arrangements, adjusting for age, on each of the individual IADL outcomes (Cox, 1970). These risk estimates were compared to those obtained when the variable of "living arrangements" was expanded to include information about the husband's health.

In those instances in which living arrangements were shown to have an independent effect on the IADL outcome, we adjusted for specific covariates. We examined the effects of each of seven sets of covariates on each of the four IADL outcomes. Those covariates found to have a significant, independent effect, adjusting for age, were included in the final model with living arrangements.

Respondents

The demographic characteristics of the interviewed cases and controls are presented in Table 4.1. Approximately 20% of the respondents were Black, reflecting the relatively large female Black population in the Detroit metropolitan area. Nationally, Black women represent about 14% of all invasive cases of breast cancer diagnosed among women aged 55 to 84 (Young et al., 1981). Nearly half of the respondents aged 65 to 84 had less than 12 years of formal education, whereas two thirds of those aged 55 to 64 reported 12 years or more. Income varied substantially with age; nearly half of those respondents aged 55 to 64 reported family income levels in excess of $25,000, whereas more than half of those in the oldest age group reported incomes of less than $10,000. Within each of the three age groups, there was no significant case–control difference by race, years of education, or 1983 self-reported family income.

RESULTS

Prevalence of IADL Problems

Housekeeping represents the most significant problem for older women with breast cancer 3 months after diagnosis (Table 4.2). Over 40% of breast cancer cases have problems completing this task. Preparing meals and grocery shop-

TABLE 4.1
Case and Control Characteristics by Age:
Detroit Metropolitan Area, 1984–1985

	Age					
	55–64 Yrs.		65–74 Yrs.		75–84 Yrs.	
	Case (N = 184) %	Control (N = 256) %	Case (N = 177) %	Control (N = 200) %	Case (N = 102) %	Control (N = 83) %
Race						
White	81.0	77.7	84.2	78.5	78.4	81.9
Black	19.0	21.1	15.3	21.0	21.6	16.9
Other	0.0	1.2	0.6	0.5	0.0	1.2
Total	100.0	100.0	100.0	100.0	100.0	100.0
Education						
Less than 12 years	31.7	32.9	50.3	51.0	57.8	49.4
12 years	37.7	42.0	31.6	35.0	19.6	25.3
More than 12 years	30.6	25.1	18.1	14.0	22.5	25.3
Total	100.0	100.0	100.0	100.0	100.0	100.0
Income (1983)	(N = 138)	(N = 214)	(N = 133)	(N = 152)	(N = 75)	(N = 60)
Less than $10,000	20.9	25.7	43.6	46.1	64.0	53.3
$10,000 - 24,999	33.3	28.0	42.9	37.5	28.0	35.0
$25,000 or more	45.8	46.3	13.5	16.4	8.0	11.7
Total	100.0	100.0	100.0	100.0	100.0	100.0

ping are considerably less problematic. Cases aged 55 to 64 and 65 to 74 are significantly more likely than controls of the same age to have problems in each of the three areas. Interestingly, there is no significant difference between cases and controls aged 75 to 84 (Table 4.3).

Marriage and Living Arrangements

There are, of course, age differences among women having different living arrangements. The proportion of married women with breast cancer declines with age, ranging from 62% for cases aged 55 to 64 to 22% for those aged 75 to 84 (Table 4.4). Conversely, the proportion of widowed women increases from 18% among those aged 55 to 64 to nearly 66% for those aged 75 to 84. Although not presented here, there is no significant difference in marital status

TABLE 4.2
Problems in the Completion of Instrumental Activities of Daily Living for Women With Breast Cancer by Age: Detroit Metropolitan Area, 1984–1985

Type	55–64 Yrs. (N = 183) %	65–74 Yrs. (N = 169) %	75–84 Yrs. (N = 98) %	Total (N = 450) %
Housekeeping				
No problem	51.6	50.6	62.4	53.6
Problem	48.4	49.4	37.6	46.4
Total	100.0	100.0	100.0	100.0
Grocery Shopping				
No problem	79.9	80.8	80.2	80.3
Problem	20.1	19.2	19.8	19.7
Total	100.0	100.0	100.0	100.0
Meal Preparation				
No problem	75.4	73.7	78.0	75.3
Problem	24.6	26.3	22.0	24.7
Total	100.0	100.0	100.0	100.0

TABLE 4.3
Problems in the Completion of Instrumental Activities of Daily Living for Breast Cancer Cases and Controls by Age: Detroit Metropolitan Area, 1984–1985

	55–64 Yrs.		65–74 Yrs.		75–84 Yrs.	
Type	Case (N = 183) %	Control (N = 256) %	Case (N = 169) %	Control (N = 199) %	Case (N = 98) %	Control (N = 81) %
Housekeeping						
No problem	51.6	67.6[a]	50.6	64.5[b]	62.4	67.5
Problem	48.4	32.4	49.4	35.5	37.6	32.5
Total	100.0	100.0	100.0	100.0	100.0	100.0
Grocery Shopping						
No problem	79.9	89.4[c]	80.8	91.5[d]	80.2	86.7
Problem	20.1	10.6	19.2	8.5	19.8	13.3
Total	100.0	100.0	100.0	100.0	100.0	100.0
Meal Preparation						
No problem	75.4	85.8[e]	73.7	87.0[f]	78.0	83.1
Problem	24.6	14.2	26.3	13.0	22.0	16.9
Total	100.0	100.0	100.0	100.0	100.0	100.0

[a]$x^2 = 11.1; p = 0.00$ [b]$x^2 = 6.2; p = 0.01$
[c]$x^2 = 7.3; p = 0.01$ [d]$x^2 = 7.7; p = 0.01$
[e]$x^2 = 7.2; p = 0.01$ [f]$x^2 = 9.2; p = 0.00$

TABLE 4.4
Marital Status for Older Women With Breast Cancer by Age:
Detroit Metropolitan Area, 1984–1985

	Age			
Marital Status*	55–64 Yrs. (N = 184) %	65–74 Yrs. (N = 177) %	75–84 Yrs. (N = 102) %	Total (N = 463) %
Never married	5.4	5.1	8.8	6.0
Married	62.0	46.3	21.6	47.1
Separated	4.3	2.3	2.0	3.0
Divorced	10.3	6.2	2.0	6.9
Widowed	17.9	40.1	65.7	36.9
TOTAL	100.0	100.0	100.0	100.0

*x^2 = 74.4; p = 0.00

between breast cancer cases and controls for any of the three age groups (p > 0.05). With regard to living arrangements, there is also an increase with age in the proportion of women with breast cancer who live alone. Nearly 57% of cases aged 75 to 84 live alone (Table 4.5). In contrast, among cases aged 55 to 64, 62% live either with their spouse or with their spouse and others. Again, these living arrangements are not unique to women with breast cancer. There is no significant difference between cases and controls in living arrangements in any of the three age groups (p > 0.05). Living arrangements were later classified into three categories: lives alone, lives with spouse, and lives with others.

Table 4.6 reports the prevalence of married women who live with an ill spouse. Of the breast cancer cases who are married, close to 32% report that

TABLE 4.5
Living Arrangements for Older Women With Breast Cancer by Age:
Detroit Metropolitan Area, 1984–1985

	Age			
Living Arrangements*	55–64 Yrs. (N = 184) %	65–74 Yrs. (N = 176) %	75–84 Yrs. (N = 102) %	Total (N = 462) %
Lives alone	18.5	37.5	56.9	34.2
Lives with spouse only	36.4	36.4	17.6	32.3
Lives with nonspouse only	13.6	10.8	17.6	13.4
Lives with spouse and others	25.5	9.1	3.9	14.5
Lives with two or more others	6.0	6.3	3.9	5.6
Total	100.0	100.0	100.0	100.0

*x^2 = 67.7; p = 0.00

TABLE 4.6
Marital Status for Older Women With Breast Cancer
by Husband's Health by Age:
Detroit Metropolitan Area, 1984–1985

	Age			
	55–64 Yrs.	65–74 Yrs.	75–84 Yrs.	Total
	(N = 184)	(N = 177)	(N = 102)	(N = 463)
Marital Status*	%	%	%	%
Single	38.0	53.7	78.4	52.9
Married,				
husband well	43.5	29.9	17.6	32.6
Married,				
husband ill	18.5	16.4	3.9	14.5
Total	100.0	100.0	100.0	100.0

*x^2 = 44.65; p = 0.00

their husbands are in ill health. Again, an ill spouse is defined by the respondent as one whose health was judged to be worse than most men his age and/or one who has been seriously ill in the past 12 months, and/or one who requires assistance in daily activities. Of the married women aged 55 to 64, 29.8% reported that their spouses were in ill heath; for those aged 65 to 74, it was 35.4%; and among those aged 75 to 84, 18.2%. There is no significant difference between cases and controls in the proportion of married women with an ill spouse ($p > 0.05$).

Living Arrangements and IADL Problems

Women with breast cancer who live alone are nearly two times more likely than patients living with a spouse to report problems in housekeeping (Table 4.7). There are no elevated risks for problems in shopping for groceries or preparing meals. Moreover, those who live with others are no more likely to report problems than those who live with their spouses.

It has been hypothesized that living alone may be especially problematic for those with a limited outside social network. Along those lines, we examined the risks of living alone for those who are socially isolated compared to those who are not (Table 4.8a & 4.8b). Following research conducted by Seeman et al. (1987), social isolation was defined as having fewer than five contacts with friends and relatives during the past month. The results indicate that housekeeping problems for women who live alone seem to be restricted to those who also are socially isolated. In contrast, those who live alone and are socially isolated are no more likely to report problems in grocery shopping and preparing meals than those who live alone and maintain more active outside social con-

TABLE 4.7
The Risk of Problems With Instrumental Activities of Daily Living
by Living Arrangements for Older Women With Breast Cancer:
Detroit Metropolitan Area, 1984–1985

Type	Odds Ratio	95% CI
Housekeeping		
Lives with spouse vs.* lives alone	1.93	(1.23, 3.02)
Lives with spouse vs. lives with others	0.99	(0.59, 1.66)
Grocery Shopping		
Lives with spouse vs. lives alone	1.32	(0.76, 2.29)
Lives with spouse vs. lives with others	1.22	(0.65, 2.29)
Meal Preparation		
Lives with spouse vs. lives alone	0.85	(0.51, 1.41)
Lives with spouse vs. lives with others	0.84	(0.51, 1.41)

*Referent category

TABLE 4.8a
The Risk of Problems With Instrumental Activities of Daily Living by
Living Arrangements for Older Women With Breast Cancer—Socially Isolated:*
Detroit Metropolitan Area, 1984–1985

Type	Odds Ratio	95% CI
Housekeeping		
Lives with spouse vs.** lives alone	2.24	(1.13, 4.45)
Lives with spouse vs. lives with others	1.06	(0.46, 2.45)
Grocery Shopping		
Lives with spouse vs. lives alone	1.54	(0.68, 3.44)
Lives with spouse vs. lives with others	1.48	(0.56, 3.91)
Meal Preparation		
Lives with spouse vs. lives alone	0.78	(0.37, 1.64)
Lives with spouse vs. lives with others	0.75	(0.30, 1.91)

*Socially Isolated = Having fewer than five social contacts with friends and relatives
during the previous month.
**Referent category.

TABLE 4.8b
The Risk of Problems With Instrumental Activities of Daily Living by Living Arrangements for Older Women With Breast Cancer— Not Socially Isolated*: Detroit Metropolitan Area, 1984–1985

Type	Odds Ratio	95% CI
Housekeeping		
Lives with spouse vs.** lives alone	1.70	(0.93, 3.11)
Lives with spouse vs. lives with others	0.93	(0.48, 1.80)
Grocery Shopping		
Lives with spouse vs. lives alone	1.13	(0.53, 2.41)
Lives with spouse vs. lives with others	1.05	(0.45, 2.43)
Meal Preparation		
Lives with spouse vs. lives alone	0.92	(0.45, 1.87)
Lives with spouse vs. lives with others	0.93	(0.43, 2.01)

*Not Socially Isolated = Having five or more social contacts with friends and relatives during the previous month.
**Referent category

tacts. The level of outside social contacts also has no effect on the risk estimates for those who live with others compared to those who live with a spouse.

The next question is whether the risk of problems in housekeeping for women living alone is due, in fact, to some other factor. To examine this issue, we adjusted for specific covariates, in this case, age, fatigue, depression, financial adequacy, and upper and lower body difficulties. These variables were found in previous analyses to be independently associated with the risk of problems with housekeeping. The results indicate that even after adjusting for these demographic, social, and physical factors, women with breast cancer who live alone are still twice as likely as those living with a spouse to have problems in this area (Table 4.9). With the exception of age at diagnosis, each of the other factors are independently associated with the risk of problems with housekeeping. It is curious that women with two or more lower body disabilities have a lower risk than that shown for women with difficulty in only one area.

Living Arrangements, the Husband's Health, and IADL Problems

Problems for women who live alone are even more apparent, when compared to those who live with a healthy spouse (Table 4.10). In addition to problems with housekeeping noted previously, the risk of problems with grocery shop-

TABLE 4.9
The Risk of Problems With Housekeeping by Living Arrangements
for Older Women With Breast Cancer, Adjusting for Selected Covariates:
Detroit Metropolitan Area, 1984–1985

	Odds Ratio	95% CI
Living Arrangements		
Lives with spouse vs.* lives alone	2.05	(1.22, 3.44)
Lives with spouse vs. lives with others	0.81	(0.44, 1.49)
Age		
55–64 yrs. vs. 65–74 yrs.	0.71	(0.43, 1.18)
55–64 yrs. vs. 75–84 yrs.	0.42	(0.22, 0.78)
Fatigue		
No vs. yes	1.62	(1.03, 2.54)
Depression		
No vs. yes	2.08	(1.22, 3.53)
Upper Body Difficulties		
0 vs. 1	1.96	(1.09, 3.53)
0 vs. 2 +	2.10	(1.22, 3.44)
Lower Body Difficulties		
0 vs. 1	2.98	(1.59, 5.56)
0 vs. 2 +	0.98	(0.53, 1.83)
Financial Adequacy		
Yes vs. no	2.23	(1.23, 4.03)

*Referent category

ping is elevated (OR = 1.94) for women who live alone, compared to those living with a healthy spouse. No elevated risk is shown for preparing meals.

Although women who live alone are at elevated risk for problems in key IADL tasks, their problems seem to be less widespread than those reported by women who live with an ill spouse. Breast cancer patients living with an ill spouse are over two times more likely than those living with a healthy spouse to report problems in each of three IADL (Table 4.10). Interestingly, those who live with others are no more likely than those living with a healthy spouse to report problems in any of the IADL tasks.

We also examined whether social isolation is associated with additional risks for women living alone or living with an ill spouse (Table 4.11a & 4.11b).

TABLE 4.10
The Risk of Problems With Instrumental Activities of Daily Living
by Living Arrangements and the Husband's Health
for Older Women With Breast Cancer:
Detroit Metropolitan Area, 1984–1985

Type	Odds Ratio	95% CI
Housekeeping		
Lives with well spouse vs.* lives alone	2.55	(1.56, 4.18)
Lives with well spouse vs. lives with others	1.31	(0.75, 2.28)
Lives with well spouse vs. lives with ill spouse	2.45	(1.34, 4.46)
Grocery Shopping		
Lives with well spouse vs. lives alone	1.94	(1.02, 3.68)
Lives with well spouse vs. lives with others	1.78	(0.87, 3.64)
Lives with well spouse vs. lives with ill spouse	2.79	(1.36, 5.75)
Meal Preparation		
Lives with well spouse vs. lives alone	1.13	(0.64, 2.00)
Lives with well spouse vs. lives with others	1.12	(0.59, 2.12)
Lives with well spouse vs. lives with ill spouse	2.29	(1.21, 4.36)

*Referent category

Among women living alone, those who are socially isolated are at an elevated risk for problems with grocery shopping. Those with outside social contacts are not. With regard to housekeeping, women who live alone are at elevated risk, regardless of the frequency of outside social contacts. The same general pattern is shown for women who live with an ill spouse. This is not the case for the risk of problems associated with preparing meals. In this case, women living with an ill spouse who are not socially isolated are at elevated risk (OR = 2.90). Those who are socially isolated are not.

After adjusting for other social and physical factors, women who live alone are two times more likely than those who live with a healthy spouse to report problems in maintaining a home (Table 4.12). The risk estimate is comparable to that found for patients living with an ill spouse. Compared to women living with a healthy spouse, those living alone are 2.6 times more likely to report difficulty with housekeeping, and for those living with an ill spouse, the risk is 2.1.

TABLE 4.11a
The Risk of Problems With Instrumental Activities of Daily Living
by Living Arrangements and the Husband's Health
for Older Women With Breast Cancer:
Socially Isolated:*
Detroit Metropolitan Area, 1984–1985

Type	Odds Ratio	95% CI
Housekeeping		
Lives with well spouse vs.** lives alone	3.03	(1.42, 6.43)
Lives with well spouse vs. lives with others	1.42	(0.58, 3.48)
Lives with well spouse vs. lives with ill spouse	2.77	(1.04, 7.38)
Grocery Shopping		
Lives with well spouse vs. lives alone	2.76	(1.03, 7.45)
Lives with well spouse vs. lives with others	2.66	(0.86, 8.21)
Lives with well spouse vs. lives with ill spouse	4.73	(1.51, 14.87)
Meal Preparation		
Lives with well spouse vs. lives alone	0.92	(0.41, 2.06)
Lives with well spouse vs. lives with others	0.88	(0.33, 2.37)
Lives with well spouse vs. lives with ill spouse	1.69	(0.62, 4.62)

*Socially Isolated = Having fewer than five social contacts with friends and relatives during the previous month.
**Referent category

TABLE 4.11b
The Risk of Problems With Instrumental Activities of Daily Living by Living Arrangements and the Husband's Health for Older Women With Breast Cancer: Not Socially Isolated:* Detroit Metropolitan Area, 1984–1985

Type	Odds Ratio	95% CI
Housekeeping		
Lives with well spouse vs.** lives alone	2.22	(1.15, 4.29)
Lives with well spouse vs. lives with others	1.22	(0.60, 2.47)
Lives with well spouse vs. lives with ill spouse	2.25	(1.05, 4.83)
Grocery Shopping		
Lives with well spouse vs. lives alone	1.45	(0.62, 3.43)
Lives with well spouse vs. lives with others	1.35	(0.53, 3.41)
Lives with well spouse vs. lives with ill spouse	1.99	(0.78, 5.11)
Meal Preparation		
Lives with well spouse vs. lives alone	1.38	(0.62, 3.10)
Lives with well spouse vs. lives with others	1.40	(0.59, 3.30)
Lives with well spouse vs. lives with ill spouse	2.90	(1.25, 6.73)

*Not Socially Isolated = Having five or more social contacts with friends and relatives during the previous month.
**Referent category

TABLE 4.12
The Risk of Problems With Housekeeping by Living Arrangements
and the Husband's Health for Older Women With Breast Cancer
Adjusting for Selected Covariates:
Detroit Metropolitan Area, 1984–1985

	Odds Ratio	95% CI
Living Arrangements		
Lives with well spouse vs.* lives alone	2.55	(1.46, 4.47)
Lives with well spouse vs. lives with others	1.02	(0.53, 1.93)
Lives with well spouse vs. lives with ill spouse	2.13	(1.06, 4.28)
Age		
55–64 yrs. vs. 65–74 yrs.	0.70	(0.42, 1.15)
55–64 yrs. vs. 75–84 yrs.	0.42	(0.22, 0.79)
Fatigue		
No vs. yes	1.63	1.03, 2.56)
Depression		
No vs. yes	1.98	(1.16, 3.39)
Upper Body Difficulties		
0 vs. 1	1.90	(1.05, 3.44)
0 vs. 2 +	2.13	(1.20, 3.79)
Lower Body Difficulties		
0 vs. 1	2.87	(1.53, 5.38)
0 vs. 2 +	0.97	(0.52, 1.79)
Financial Adequacy		
Yes vs. no	2.14	(1.18, 3.88)

*Referent category

In contrast, there is no elevated risk for problems associated with preparing meals or grocery shopping reported by women with breast cancer who live alone, compared to those living with a healthy spouse (Tables 4.13 and 4.14). There is some evidence to suggest, however, that women with an ill spouse are more likely to have problems in these areas. The risk estimates for these women approach, but do not attain, statistical significance. Reduced upper and lower body strength, auditory difficulty, and reports of depression are associated most strongly with difficulties in these areas.

TABLE 4.13
The Risk of Problems With Grocery Shopping by Living Arrangements
and the Husband's Health for Older Women With Breast Cancer
Adjusting for Selected Covariates:
Detroit Metropolitan Area, 1984–1985

	Odds Ratio	95% CI
Living Arrangements		
Lives with well spouse vs.* lives alone	1.48	(0.74, 2.97)
Lives with well spouse vs. lives with others	1.11	(0.49, 2.32)
Lives with well spouse vs. lives with ill spouse	2.06	(0.94, 4.52)
Age		
55–64 yrs. vs. 65–74 yrs.	0.71	(0.39, 1.32)
55–64 yrs. vs. 75–84 yrs.	0.88	(0.43, 1.81)
Depression		
No vs. yes	2.80	(1.63, 4.81)
Lower Body Difficulties		
0 vs. 1	2.04	(1.01, 4.13)
0 vs. 2 +	3.66	(2.01, 6.69)

*Referent category

DISCUSSION

Living arrangements are associated with the risk of problems for older women with breast cancer in completing selected IADL tasks. Unlike studies of older people in the general population (Magaziner et al., 1988), our results suggest that living alone for women newly diagnosed with breast cancer is associated with an elevated risk for problems with housekeeping, especially for those women with limited outside social contacts. The results also indicate, at least for this IADL task, that living arrangements and physical disabilities, such as difficulty in upper and lower body tasks, are each associated with reported problems. On the other hand, problems with less strenuous tasks such as shopping for groceries and preparing meals are associated with reported depression and levels of physical functioning, but not with living arrangements.

It is also important to note that women with breast cancer who live with people, other than a spouse, are no more likely to have difficulty than women who live with a spouse. This seems to suggest that assistance to complete the

TABLE 4.14
The Risk of Problems With Meal Preparation by Living Arrangements
and the Husband's Health for Older Women With Breast Cancer
Adjusting for Selected Covariates:
Detroit Metropolitan Area, 1984–1985

	Odds Ratio	95% CI
Living Arrangements		
Lives with well spouse vs.* lives alone	0.82	(0.45, 1.69)
Lives with well spouse vs. lives with others	0.66	(0.29, 1.30)
Lives with well spouse vs. lives with ill spouse	2.05	(0.96, 4.36)
Age		
55–64 yrs. vs. 65–74 yrs.	0.78	(0.44, 1.34)
55–64 yrs. vs. 75–84 yrs.	0.52	(0.24, 1.12)
Depression		
No vs. yes	2.07	(1.20, 3.60)
Lower Body Difficulties		
0 vs. 1	2.44	(1.24, 4.80)
0 vs. 2 +	3.73	(1.91, 7.32)
Upper Body Difficulties		
0 vs. 1	2.55	(1.14, 5.67)
0 vs. 2 +	2.78	(1.30, 5.96)
Hearing Acuity		
Good/Excellent vs. Fair/Poor	2.42	(1.34, 4.36)

*Referent category

daily tasks of housekeeping, meal preparation, and grocery shopping can be obtained from household members other than a spouse.

The results also indicate that living with a spouse is not always beneficial; the husband's health is clearly an important factor in dealing with everyday tasks. Those women who live with a healthy spouse are least likely to report problems in any of the IADL tasks. For those living with an ill spouse, however, the problems are at least as serious as those facing women who live alone. There are a number of possible explanations. For a woman recuperating from breast cancer and, in most cases, major surgery, a husband in poor health may represent an added burden. It may mean that she must care for her husband while trying to cope with her own condition. Moreover, her husband may not represent a source of tangible support in housekeeping, grocery shopping, and preparing meals.

Although these results are interesting and have implications for understanding the effects of social relations for adjustment following breast cancer, more detailed analyses are required. We recommend that research strategies be developed along the following lines:

1. The significance of living arrangements and the husband's health for subgroups of women with breast cancer should be further explored. The health status of single people compared to married people has been shown in other studies to be related to the age of the population. An ill spouse may be more problematic for women in their 50s than it is for women in their 70s. Likewise, the effects may vary by degree of isolation, level of disability, and stage of disease at diagnosis. The systematic study of interaction effects will require a larger sample. In our own project, we have recently completed interviews with a new cohort of cases and controls. Younger women aged 40 to 54 also have been included so that functioning could be investigated across a broader age spectrum. The final sample will include over 1,000 women with breast cancer and 1,000 women without the disease aged 40 to 84.

2. Research should be conducted to examine the effects of marital status and living arrangements over a longer period of time. In the next phase of the analysis, we examine the risk of problems in IADL tasks 12 months after diagnosis. To determine to what extent these social factors affect the risk of death following diagnosis also will be worthwhile. Along these lines, it also will be important to determine to what extent living arrangements are affected by the diagnosis and treatment of the breast cancer itself. Are those women who live alone likely to stay with friends and relatives or have others stay with them during the period immediately following the surgery for breast cancer? It is also necessary to examine the effects of living arrangements in women with breast cancer compared to women of the same age without the disease. This is necessary to investigate directly whether living alone or living with an ill spouse is especially problematic for women newly diagnosed and treated with a serious health problem.

3. It is important to examine in greater detail the effects of outside social contacts for women who either live alone or live with an ill spouse. Although there is some suggestion that limited outside social contacts are associated with housekeeping problems for cases who live alone, the effects of outside social contacts seem inconsistent for other IADL tasks. Alternative measures of social networks should be considered.

4. More sophisticated assessments of the husband's health should be made. In addition to the wife's assessment, it is necessary to interview the husband. Direct assessments of health also should be conducted, including the number and type of health problems and disabilities. We also should determine in greater detail how the husband's health affects the completion of IADL tasks. This will help to clarify to what extent an ill spouse represents an added burden and to what extent the husband represents a lost source of social support. Along these lines, it is necessary to investigate in greater detail the prevalence and effects of caregiving among older women newly diagnosed with breast cancer.

5. Other functional outcomes should be identified. Our analysis focused on IADL outcomes because of their significance for measuring activities necessary for indepen-

dent living. For younger women, marital status and living arrangements may be associated with problems in returning to work or with childcare.

In conclusion, the investigation of marital status and living arrangements, and especially the impact of the husband's health, may provide useful information in explaining why some women with breast cancer do well following diagnosis and treatment, whereas others do not. With this information, it may be possible to design special interventions for breast cancer patients who either live alone or live with an ill spouse.

ACKNOWLEDGMENT

Research was supported through NIA grant (R01-AG04969), NCI contract (NO1 CN-55423), and by the United Foundation of Detroit.

REFERENCES

Berkman, L. F. (1985). The relationship of social networks and social support to morbidity and mortality. In S. Cohen & S. L. Syme (Eds.), *Social support and health* (pp. 241–261). New York: Academic Press.

Bloom, J. R., Ross, R., & Burnell, G. (1978). The effect of social support on patient adjustment after breast surgery. *Patient Counseling and Health Education, 1,* 50–59.

Branch, L. G. (1984). Relative risk rates of nonmedical predictors of institutional care among the elderly. *Comprehensive Therapy, 10,* 33–40.

Branch, L. G. (1988). Applications of epidemiological research in aging to planning and policy: The Massachusetts Health Care Panel Study. In J. Brody & G. L. Maddox (Eds.), *Epidemiology and Aging* (pp. 177–188). New York: Springer.

Branch, L. G., & Jette, A. M. (1981). Framingham disability study: I. Social disability among the aging. *American Journal of Public Health, 71,* 1202–1210.

Branch, L. G., & Jette, A. M. (1982). A prospective study of long-term care institutionalization among the aged. *American Journal of Public Health, 72,* 1373–1379.

Cafferata, G. L. (1987). Marital status, living arrangements, and the use of health services by elderly persons. *Journal of Gerontology, 42,* 613–618.

Commonwealth Fund Commission on Elderly People Living Alone. (1987, April 16). *Old, alone, and poor: A plan for reducing poverty among elderly people living alone.* Baltimore, MD: Author.

Cox, D. R. (1970). *The analysis of binary data.* London: Methuen.

DiMatteo, M., & Hays, R. (1981). Social support and serius illness. In B. Gottlieb (Ed.), *Social networks and social support* (pp. 117–148). Beverly Hills, CA: Sage.

Fengler, A. P., & Goodrich, N. (1979). Wives of elderly disabled men: The hidden patients. *The Gerontologist, 19,* 175.

Gilford, D. M. (Ed.). (1988). *The aging population in the twenty-first century: Statistics for health policy.* Washington, DC: National Academy Press.

Horowitz, A. (1985). Family caregiving to the frail elderly. *Annual Review of Gerontology and Geriatrics, 5,* 194–246.

Kane, R .A. (1983). Coordination of cancer treatment and social support for the elderly. In R. Yancik, P. Carbone, W. B. Patterson, K. Steel, & W. D. Terry (Eds.), *Perspectives on prevention and treatment of cancer in the elderly* (pp. 227–238). New York: Raven Press.

Kane, R. A., & Kane, R. L. (1987). *Long-term care: Principles, programs, and policies.* New York: Springer.

Kavesh, W. N. (1986). Home care: Process, outcome, cost. *Annual Review of Gerontology and Geriatrics, 6,* 135–195.

Lawton, M. P. (1972). Assessing the competence of older people. In D. Kent, R. Kastenbaum, & S. Sherwood (Eds.), *Research planning and action for the elderly* (pp. 122–143). New York: Behavioral.

Magaziner, J., Cadigan, D. A., Hebel, J. R., & Parry, R. E. (1988). Health and living arrangements among older women: does living alone increase the risk of illness? *Journal of Gerontology: Medical Sciences, 43,* M127–133.

Moritz, D. J., Kasl, S. V., & Berkman, L. F. (1989). The health impact of living with a cognitively impaired elderly spouse: depressive symptoms and social functioning. *Journal of Gerontology: Social Sciences, 44,* S17–27.

Ortmeyer, C. F. (1974). Variations in mortality, morbidity, and health care by marital status. In L.L Erhardt & J. E. Berlin (Eds.), *Mortality and morbidity in the United States* (pp. 159–184). Cambridge, MA: Harvard University Press.

Ries, L. F., Pollack, E. S., & Young, J. L. (1983). Cancer patient survival: Surveillance, epidemiology, and end results program, 1973–79. *Journal of the National Cancer Institute, 70,* 693–707.

Rubinstein, R. L. (1984). The elderly who live alone and their social supports. *Annual Review of Gerontology and Geriatrics, 4,* 165–193.

Satariano, W. A., Ragheb, N. E., Branch, L. G., & Swanson, G. M. (1990). Difficulties in physical functioning reported by middle-aged and elderly women with breast cancer: A case–control comparison. *Journal of Gerontology: Medical Sciences, 45,* M3–11.

Satariano, W. A., Ragheb, N. E., Buck, K. A., Swanson, G. M., & Branch, L. G. (1989). Aging and breast cancer: A case–control comparison of instrumental functioning. *Journal of Aging and Health, 1,* 209–233.

Satariano, W. A., Ragheb, N. E., & DuPuis, M. H. (1989). Comorbidity in older women with breast cancer: an epidemiologic approach. In R. Yancik & J. Yates (Eds.), *Cancer in the elderly: Approaches to early detection and treatment* (pp. 73–106). New York: Springer.

Seeman, T. E., Kaplan, G. A., Knudsen, L., Cohen, R., & Guralnik, J. (1987). Social network ties and mortality among the elderly in the Alameda County study. *American Journal of Epidemiology, 126,* 714–723.

Siegel, J., & Davidson, M. (1984). Demographic and socioeconomic aspects of aging in the United States. In *Current population reports* (Special Studies Series P-23, No. 138). Washington, DC: U.S. Department of Commerce.

Sondik, E., Young, J. L., Horm, J., & Ries, L. G. (1988). *1987 annual cancer statistics review.* Bethesda, MD: National Institutes of Health.

Taylor, S. E., Lichtman, R. R., Wood, J. V., Bluming, A.Z, Dosik, G. M., & Leibowitz, R. L. (1985). Illness-related and treatment-related factors in psychological adjustment to breast cancer. *Cancer, 55,* 2506–2513.

Thomas, S. G. (1978). Breast cancer: The psychosocial issues. *Cancer Nursing, 1,* 53–60.

Verbrugge, L. M. (1979). Marital status and health. *Journal of Marriage and the Family, 42,* 267–285.

Vinokur, A. D., Threatt, B. A., Vinokur-Kaplan, D., & Satariano, W. A. (1990). The process of recovery from breast cancer for younger and older patients: Changes during the first year. *Cancer, 65,* 1242–1254.

Wortman, C. B., & Conway, T. L. (1985). The role of social support in adaptation and recovery from physical illness. In S. Cohen & S. L. Syme, *Social support and health* (pp. 281–302). New York: Academic Press.

Young, J. L., Percy, C., & Asire, A. (Eds.). (1981). *Surveillance, epidemiology, and end results*. Bethesda, MD: National Institutes of Health.

Zarit, S. H., Todd, P. A., Zarit, J. M. (1986). Subjective burden of husbands and wives as caregivers: A longitudinal study. *The Gerontologist, 26*, 260–266.

The Content and Context
of Effective Spousal Support

Sheldon Cohen
Carnegie Mellon University

Satariano and Ragheb's analysis of adjustment to breast cancer in chapter 4 indicates that married women adjust better than nonmarried women *except* when their husbands are ill. Those with ill husbands indicate levels of adjustment that are equivalent to their nonmarried counterparts. These data qualify the generally accepted notion that marriage improves health and well-being and draw attention to the importance of the context of marital relationships in determining whether they are health promoting. This discussion expands on this issue by attempting to delineate types of spousal behaviors and behavioral contexts that result in effective spousal support.

Our own work is concerned with specifying the conditions under which spouses are effective supporters of health-promoting behaviors. Here, we discuss a microanalytic study of spousal behaviors performed in response to an attempt to quit smoking cigarettes and maintain abstinence from smoking. In short, we measure spousal behaviors that are characterized by cooperation and reinforcement (positive) or by nagging and policing (negative) and assess their role in successful quitting. We also view the effectiveness of these behaviors in the context of one another (positive/negative behaviors) as well as in the context of how persons quitting smoking expect their spouses to behave. We raise three questions in this regard: (a) How important are the mere frequencies of positive (supportive) and negative (nonsupportive) behaviors? (b) Is the effectiveness of the frequency of supportive behaviors influenced by the frequency of nonsupportive ones? (c) Is the effectiveness of support one receives influenced by the support one expects?

METHODS

Subjects.   The subjects were 221 persons making a serious attempt to quit smoking by themselves. In order to qualify for participation, a subject needed to be 18 or older, smoke at least 10 cigarettes a day, and have not yet begun the quitting process. The mean number of cigarettes smoked at baseline was 26.8 and the mean years as a smoker was 23.3. Of the subjects, 70% were female and the mean age was 40.

Interviews

Those meeting study criteria were given a baseline interview approximately 1 month prior to initiating quit attempts, and follow-up interviews 1, 2, 3, 6, and 12 months after their expected quit dates.

Assessing Spousal Behavior.   The *first* 145 of the 221 subjects were administered a measure of expected partner support for quitting smoking at baseline, while all 221 were administered a measure of received partner support for quitting at 1 month. (The baseline support measure was replaced with a questionnaire addressing another issue at mid study.)

Both expected and received partner support were assessed with the 20-item version of the Partner Interaction Questionnaire (PIQ-20). The PIQ-20 is a self-report questionnaire assessing the specific behaviors that spouse or romantic partner perform in response to a person's attempts to quit smoking (Cohen & Lichtenstein, 1990; Mermelstein, Lichtenstein, & McIntyre, 1983). At base-line, before subjects started the quitting process, we asked for an indication of behaviors that were *expected* from partners. At 1-month follow-up we asked for indication of behaviors actually *received* from the partner. For each item, subjects indicate the frequency of each expected or received behavior on a 5-point scale: (0) never; (1) almost never; (2) sometimes; (3) fairly often; and (4) very often.

The PIQ-20 includes separate 10-item subscales assessing positive and nega-tive behaviors. The positive behaviors are characterized by cooperation and reinforcement for the quitting attempt and the negative behaviors by nagging and policing. Examples from the positive behavior subscale include (a) com-pliment you on not smoking, (b) congratulate you for your decision to quit smoking, and (c) help you think of substitutes for smoking. Examples from the negative behavior subscale include (a) comment that smoking is a dirty habit, (b) talk you out of smoking a cigarette, and (c) comment on your lack of willpower. Three scores are derived from the PIQ: (1) frequency of positive behaviors, (2) frequency of negative behaviors, and (3) ratio of positive to nega-tive behaviors.

Assessing Smoking Status. All of the interviews included detailed assessment of smoking status. *Point-prevalence abstinence* at a panel was assigned to persons who said that they were not currently smoking and had not smoked "even a puff" during the last week. *Continuous abstinence* was assigned to persons who were point-prevalent abstinent at all follow-up interviews up to the point of assessment (e.g., at 1 and 3 months for 3 months of continuous abstinence) and had not smoked more than three days since quitting.

Biochemical Verification. At each interview, subjects were reminded that at some as yet unscheduled point of the study, the investigators would biochemically verify their smoking status. All persons who reported abstinence at 6 months were scheduled for verification with both CO and saliva cotinine. All persons continuously abstinent at 6 months were tested and all had CO and cotinine levels consistent with their continuous abstinence status.

RESULTS

PIQ Mean Scores

For both positive and negative behaviors, subjects received a lower frequency of behaviors than they expected. Mean positive behavior scores were 28.70 on the expected scale and 21.08 on the received scale [$t(144)$ = 9.04, $p <$ .001]. Mean negative behavior scores were 17.35 on the expected scale and 13.07 on the received scale [$t(144)$ = 5.70, $p <$ .001]. For the ratio of positive to negative behaviors, subjects had a higher received ratio (3.57) than they expected [2.60; $t(144)$ = 2.18, $p <$ .03]. The correlations between expected and received scores were .41 (df = 144, $p <$ .001) for positive behaviors, .45 (df = 144, $p <$ .001) for negative behaviors, and .22 (df = 144, $p <$ .007) for the positive/negative ratio.

Males and females differed only on the ratios of positive/negative scores. Females both expected and received a larger ratio of positive to negative behaviors than males. The mean expected male ratio was 2.06, whereas the mean expected female ratio was 3.36 [$t(194)$ = 2.95, $p <$ .004]. Similarly, the mean received male ratio was 2.70, whereas the received female ratio was 4.08 [$t(167)$ = 2.03, $p <$ .04].

Abstinence Rates

At 1 month, 10.4% of the sample (23 of 221) were continuously abstinent. There is relatively little change in the percent of persons continuously abstinent at subsequent follow-ups (only 12 relapsing between 1 and 12 months:

6.8% [15 of 219] abstinent at 3 months, 5.5% [12 of 218] at 6 months, and 5% [11 of 219] at 12 months) and hence prospective lag prediction of relapse (e.g., predicting relapse from 1- to 3-month follow-ups) was not possible. These rates are consistent with those reported in other studies of self-quitters (e.g., median of 4.2% at 12 months for five studies reported by Cohen et al., 1989).

Predicting Continuous Abstinence

Each of the primary outcome analyses is a logistic regression. The dichotomous variable abstinent/smoking is regressed on various combinations of PIQ scale scores. Abstinence is coded as "1" and smoking as "0." The probability values we report are based on treating the regression coefficient divided by its standard error as a t value and using two-tailed tests (Dixon, 1985). In order to illustrate the nature of effects indicated by significant coefficients, we report percent abstinence for persons high (above the median) and low (below the median) on a variable.

We do separate analyses of continuous abstinence at 1, 3, 6, and 12 months post quit date. Analyses of the same variable at different panels are not independent (e.g., the people abstinent at 12 months were abstinent at all previous panels). The purpose of presenting data from each successive panel is to determine the predictive ability of the partner support in relation to an *increasingly conservative* outcome criterion.

The first set of equations is designed to test the independent influences of the *frequencies* of positive and negative received behaviors on abstinence. The second set is designed to test whether the ratio of positive/negative behaviors will predict continuous abstinence. Finally, we conduct a set of conservative analyses to determine whether associations between the ratio and outcomes occur above and beyond the influence of positive and negative behavior frequencies. Because of the multiple tests, we use a conservative alpha of $p < .01$ to evaluate these hypotheses. Findings at the $p < .05$ level are viewed as suggestive but not conclusive.

Received Support

The Independent Effects of Positive and Negative Behaviors. In a single equation, abstinence/smoking was regressed on the number of positive behaviors received ($+R$) and the number of negative behaviors received ($-R$). The more positive behaviors one received, the *more* likely they were to be continuously abstinent at 1 month (5.1% abstinence for persons low on $+R$ and 16.3% for those high on $+R$, $p < .01$). A similar suggestive effect occurred at 3 months (4.2% for low $+R$ and 9.8% for high $+R$, $p < .05$) but there were no relations between positive behaviors and abstinence at 6- and 12-month follow-ups. There was also a suggestive association between the frequency of negative behaviors and abstinence at 1 month. The more negative behaviors, the *less* likely they were to be continuously abstinent (12.5% for low $-R$ and 8.3% for those high on $-R$). There were no associations between frequency of negative behaviors and any of the subsequent follow-ups.

The Proportion of Positive to Negative Behaviors.   A set of analyses was conducted to determine whether the *ratio* of positive to negative behaviors received ($+R/-R$) predicted continuous abstinence. The first logistic regression included only the ratio $+R/-R$. The ratio is associated with continuous abstinence at the 1-, 3-, 6-, and 12-month follow-ups ($p < .01$ for all). As summarized in Fig. 1, in all cases, the greater the proportion of positive to negative behaviors the greater the abstinence rate. In order to determine whether the ratio accounted for variance in abstinence above and beyond that accounted for by $+R$ and $-R$, a third regression was run including all three variables, $+R$, $-R$, and $+R/-R$, as predictors. Even after partialing out the constituent parts of the ratio, there is a suggestive relation ($p < .05$) between the proportion $+R/-R$ and continuous abstinence at 1, 6, and 12 months. The coefficient at 3 months was marginally ($p < .07$) significant. Again, in all cases, the higher the frequency of positive relative to negative behaviors, the greater

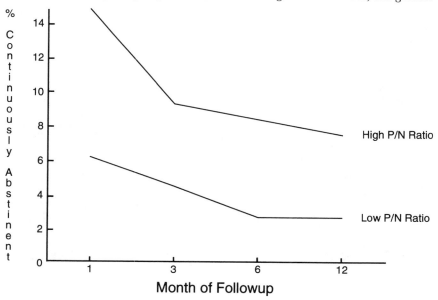

FIG. 1. Percent persons continuously abstinent at each panel as a function of the ratio of positive/negative behaviors received from their spouse or partner.

the probability of being abstinent. The positive behavior score was marginally predictive at 1 month ($p < .05$), but neither positive nor negative behavior coefficients were significant at any other time in equations where the ratio was included.

Expected Support

Our concern with expected partner support was driven by an interest in the influence of expected support on the effectiveness of received support. Although there were indications of expectations influencing the effectiveness of received support, none of the critical analyses reached statistical significance. The most interesting distribution of proportions is presented in Fig. 2. These data suggest that persons with higher positive to negative behavior ratios than they expected are more likely to be abstinent than those getting what they expected and those with lower positive to negative behavior ratios than they expected. We attribute the lack of significant effects to the smaller sample size for persons receiving the expected PIQ at baseline. There were similarly no independent effects of expectation on abstinence.

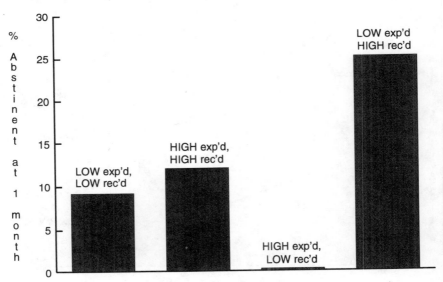

FIG. 2. Percent persons abstinent at 1 month as a function of the ratio of positive/negative behaviors they expected from their spouse or partner and the ratio of positive/negative behaviors they received.

Relation of PIQ to Partner Relationship and Gender

A series of analyses of variance was conducted in order to determine whether any of the expected or received PIQ scores were related to whether the named partner was a spouse or not, the gender of the smoker, and the smoking status of the partner. There were no differences on any PIQ score on any of these criteria.

DISCUSSION

Let us return to the three questions raised earlier in this chapter regarding the nature and context of behaviors that support spouses.

How Important are the Mere Frequencies of Positive and Negative Behaviors?

Mere frequency appears to be of little importance. Frequency of positive behaviors alone predicts only 1-month abstinence and none of the associations between negative behaviors and abstinence reached the $p < .01$ criterion.

Is the Effectiveness of the Frequency of Supportive Behaviors Influenced by the Frequency of Nonsupportive Ones?

The ratio of positive/negative behaviors as perceived by the quitter is the best predictor of abstinence. The ratio predicts continuous abstinence through 12 months. Moreover, suggestive ($p < .05$) effects remained even after a very conservative analysis partialing out variance accounted for by the frequency of positive and negative behaviors. Hence, it appears that the frequency of spousal positive behaviors is interpreted in the context of the frequency of negative ones. It is possible that people generate a sense of supportiveness based on the *relative* frequency of positive to negative behaviors and this is what is associated with continuous success in quitting.

Is the Effectiveness of Support One Receives Influenced by the Support One Expects?

It appears that subjects' support expectancies were reasonable but not particularly accurate. They received fewer positive and negative behaviors than expected, and received a higher positive to negative ratio than expected. In short, their partners were less interactive in regard to their quitting than they expected, but relatively more of the interactions were positive in nature.

Our data in regard to how expectancies influence the effectiveness of received support are merely suggestive. They do, however, indicate the possibility that the receipt of more positive relative to negative behaviors than expected may maximally influence quitting and maintenance. These effects might reach statistical significance with a larger sample size (only 145 were available for these analyses as opposed to 221 for the received support analyses).

Summary

In summary, our study indicates the importance of the content and context of spousal behaviors in supporting health behavior change. We think that microanalytic studies of behavioral interchanges between spouses will help clarify what behaviors are interpreted as supportive, what behaviors improve health and well-being, and the conditions under which supportive behaviors are most effective. Such work will provide a better basic view of the spousal support process as well as aid in the design and implementation of social support interventions.

ACKNOWLEDGMENTS

Detailed description of the study and data analyses presented in this chapter are reported in Cohen and Lichtenstein (1990). Preparation of this article was supported by a Research Scientist Development Award from the National Institute of Mental Health to the first author (K02 MH00721). Research reported in this article was supported by a grant from the National Cancer Institute (CA38243).

REFERENCES

Cohen, S., & Lichtenstein, E. (1990). Partner behavior that supports quitting smoking. *Journal of Consulting and Clinical Psychology, 58*, 304–309.
Cohen, S., Lichtenstein, E., Prochaska, J. O., Rossi, J., Gritz, E. R., Carr, C. R., Orleans, C. T., Schoenbach, V. J., Biener, L., Abrams, D., DiClemente, C., Curry, S., Marlat, G. A., Cummings, K. M., Emont, S. L., Giovino, G., & Ossip-Klein, D. (1989). Debunking myths about self-quitting: Evidence from 10 prospective studies of persons who quit smoking by themselves. *American Psychologist, 44*, 1355–1365.
Dixon, W. J., (Ed.). (1985). *BMDP Statistical Software manual*. Berkeley, CA: University of California Press.
Mermelstein, R., Lichtenstein, E., & McIntyre, K. (1983). Partner support and relapse in smoking cessation programs. *Journal of Consulting and Clinical Psychology, 51*, 465–466.

Reducing Disability in Research

Adrian M. Ostfeld
Yale University School of Medicine

Because much of the meaning and value of research in this area is linked with the stability variability of IADL, the question that arises first concerns the stability of these self-reports. Disability as a result of arthritic disease may vary from hour to hour. Clinical experience suggests that elderly are more likely to feel and report disability in cold weather. Very little work has been done on the variability of measures of functional deficit (Hazzard, Andres, Bierman, & Blass, 1989). In subsequent research much could be added by remeasuring disability.

Certain decisions about inclusion and classification of data need to be reconsidered. For instance, why were household members under 18 excluded from data collection? Certainly young adults and children can provide help to disabled elders. To discount them may inflate the interpretation of the value of assistance from adults in the household. Similarly persons living with spouse were placed into one group and those living with spouse and others—without regard for the number, age and help received from others—were placed into another group. This distinction obscures interpretation of results. Another household member besides the spouse can provide help. An ill spouse can be compensated for by a helpful other.

The method of assessment of health of husband requires additional thought. A wife's rating of her husband's health may reflect the pessimism of depression. Husband's hospitalization here interpreted to mean poor health, may indicate improvement or cure.

As is frequently written, the Achilles heel of the case–control study is selection of the control group. In this study, too, there are important differences between cases and controls that may influence the results of the study. Aside from presence or absence of breast cancer, cases and controls differ in several ways. The cases have had surgery that in some cases requires removal of chest muscles and that may induce hurts to feminine image and to self-esteem. The cases are also more likely to have had anemia, fever, postoperative pain, debilitating cancer chemotherapy, diabetic nerve and muscle disease, and adiposity. Discussion of the protocol with a physician in the pilot stage can help ameliorate this kind of problem.

In addition to these specific concerns, certain generic issues need to be raised. Are we trying to quantitate processes that are too subtle, too complex and too interrelated to be quantified? We count things and give them names. Are we counting the right things and using the right units of measurement? I am troubled by the fact that we do not usually include love in our attempts to measure quality of life. And what a powerful effect it may have. We get at love indirectly when we assess social networks and social supports but the crucial word and the crucial feeling are not asked about. We should begin to do so.

Although it is not difficult to identify improvements needed in such research, it is also apparent that the work has considerable value. In the area in which the data were collected, they are a guide to planning, policy and action. They help discharge planners, hospital social workers, Visiting Nurses Associations, home-care agencies, HMOs, and those physicians who will listen and learn use the knowledge to improve the quality and perhaps the duration of life for women and families in a tough spot. They help determine health policy, the allocation of resources, and promote humane legislation.

Although it is unlikely that exactly the same relationships would obtain at another site, they alert investigators everywhere about what to look for and how to go about organizing the look. As the literature matures, we learn what factors are site-specific and what are general. And this helps the action personnel I have listed here, contribute to clearer comprehension of the needs of people in trouble and to both understanding and improving the human condition. That is enough for me.

REFERENCES

Hazzard, W. R., Andres, R., Bierman, E. L., & Blass, J. P. (Eds.). (1989). *Principles of geriatric medicine and gerontology* (2nd ed.). New York: McGraw Hill.

Social Factors and the Onset and Outcome of Depression

Linda K. George
Duke University

A majority of current research designed to inform us about the older population focuses on individual differences. In these studies, it is typical to obtain data from a sample that represents the older population in total or in part. It also is common in such studies to adopt and/or adapt theories previously tested on samples of younger and middle-aged adults—or on the adult population as a whole—and to determine the degree to which those theories also are able to explain individual differences among older adults.

Studies of the relationships between social factors and depression are a case in point. A large number of previous studies testify to the relationships between social factors—particularly demographic characteristics, social stress (variously measured as life events, chronic stress, and daily hassles), and social support (appropriately measured multidimensionally)—and depression. Space limitations preclude a review of those studies. For the purposes at hand, however, we should note that this research base includes both studies based on samples of adults of all ages (e.g., Burks & Martin, 1985; Cronkite & Moos, 1984; DeLongis, Coyne, Dakof, Folkman, & Lazarus, 1982; Dohrenwend, 1973; Dressler, 1985; Kanner, Coyne, Schaefer, & Lazarus, 1981; Kaplan, Robins, & Martin, 1983; Kessler, 1979; Kessler & McLeod, 1985; Lin & Ensel, 1984; Lin, Simeone, Ensel, & Kuo, 1979; Lin, Woelfel, & Light, 1985; Monroe, 1983; Turner, 1981; Wethington & Kessler, 1986; Wheaton, 1983; Williams, Ware, & Donald, 1981; Zarski, 1984) and studies based on samples of older adults (e.g., Dimond, Lund, & Caserta, 1987; Holahan & Holahan, 1987; Holahan, Holahan, & Belk, 1984; Krause, 1986, 1987a, 1987b, 1987c; Norris & Murrell, 1984).

In spite of this large base of previous research, relatively few studies focus on the role of age in the relationships between social factors and depression. To be sure, most studies include age as an independent or control variable— and this is the case whether the samples include adults of all ages or are restricted to older adults. But determining whether age has a significant main effect on depression is but part of the story. It also is possible that age interacts with social factors, moderating their effects on depression. The potential importance of age interactions needs to be recognized. Age interactions suggest that the meaning and/or salience of social factors vary across age or stage in the life course.

The purpose of this chapter is to explore the interactions of age with social factors as they affect both the onset of and recovery from depression. Two studies are reported. The first is an epidemiologic study of a representative sample of community-dwelling adults and examines interactions of age and social factors as they affect the onset of major depression. The second is a clinical study of depressed adults. In this study, we examine interactions of age and social factors as they affect recovery from major depression.

STUDY 1: AGE, SOCIAL FACTORS, AND THE ONSET OF MAJOR DEPRESSION

Although consensus remains out of reach, studies of the social antecedents of psychiatric disorders increasingly focus on several specific categories of independent variables. In a previous review, I suggested that six categories of social variables are suggested by previous research (George, 1989). First, virtually all studies include *demographic variables* that index differential risk of specific psychiatric disorders. Examples of the demographic variables included in previous studies include age, gender, and race. In spite of substantial evidence that demographic variables are statistically related to psychiatric disorder, the mechanisms that underlie these relationships remain unclear. Second, *early events and achievements* are often hypothesized to have persisting effects on vulnerability to psychiatric disorders. Examples of such variables include childhood traumas (e.g., early parental death or divorce) and educational attainment. Third, *later events and achievements* also are commonly examined as predictors of psychiatric morbidity. Examples of these factors include marital status and/or history, current occupation, and income.

Fourth, *social integration* has been hypothesized by some investigators to be a meaningful antecedent of psychiatric disorder—although there is probably less consensus about this category than about the other five. The term *social integration* is used in two primary ways in previous research. Some investigators focus on social integration at the individual level, referring to individuals' attachments to social structure (e.g., religious and voluntary organization participation). Other investigators focus on social integration at the aggregate level, referring to levels of social organization versus disorganization in the environment. Such researchers are likely to examine aggregate variables such as neighborhood stability and other indicators of social organization. Fifth are what Brown and Harris (1978) refer to as *vulnerability and protective factors*, which refer to relatively stable assets and liabilities that can alter the risk of psychiatric morbidity. In this area, chronic stress (presumably a vulnerability factor) and social support (a presumed protective factor) are most commonly examined. Finally, are *coping efforts* and what Brown and Harris (1978) refer to as *provoking agents*. Examples of variables representing this category include specific coping strategies and stressful life events. Coping efforts and, especially, provoking agents are viewed as less stable than vulnerability and protective factors. Undoubtedly some investigators would classify the hypothesized social antecedents of mental illness differently than above. Nonetheless, most recent studies include several of these categories of independent variables in their predictions of psychiatric disorder.

Two design issues that bifurcate previous studies of the social antecedents of psychiatric disorder also merit brief attention. First, most studies rely on measures of psychiatric symptoms and few attempt to measure psychiatric disorders in diagnostic terms compatible with current psychiatric nomenclature (i.e., American Psychiatric Association, 1980, 1987). It is not clear whether results based on symptom scales differ substantially from those based on diagnostic measures. It is clear, however, that studies relying on symptom scales cannot be used to predict the onset of psychiatric disorders (i.e., incident cases). Indeed, to my knowledge, there are no previous studies of the social antecedents of incident cases of psychiatric disorder in representative community populations. (Studies by Brown and Harris, 1978, and by Henderson, 1981, come very close to this, but do not operationalize psychiatric disorders using the nomenclature of clinical psychiatry.) Second, some studies of the predictors of psychiatric disorders are based on cross-sectional data and others are based on longitudinal data. Obviously, longitudinal data are preferable and, fortunately, are more common among recent studies.

In this study, 10 factors that previous research suggests may be implicated in the onset of depression are examined: age, gender, race, urban versus rural residence, marital status, education, income, physical illnesses, stressful life events, and subjective perceptions of social support. The dependent variable is a diagnostic measure of major depression, as defined in DSM-III (American Psychiatric Association, 1980). In addition, the model is applied longitudinally with predictors typically measured prior to the onset of major depression. Initially, a multivariate model is presented that examines the main effects of the 10 risk factors on onset of major depression. Subsequently, interactions between age and the other nine risk factors are examined.

Sample

The data used in this study are from the Duke University Epidemiologic Catchment Area (ECA) Project. The ECA Program is a multi-site collaborative study of psychiatric disorders sponsored by the National Institute of Mental Health. Five universities participated in the ECA Program, surveying defined local populations consisting of one or more Community Mental Health Center catchment areas: Yale University, surveying greater New Haven; Johns Hopkins University, surveying East Baltimore; Washington University, surveying greater St. Louis; Duke University, surveying the Piedmont region of North Carolina; and UCLA, surveying East Los Angeles and Venice. All the data reported here are from the Duke University ECA project.

The geographic area sampled in the Duke University ECA Project consisted of five counties in north central North Carolina. The sample is about evenly split between one urban county (i.e., defined as part of a SMSA by the U.S. Bureau of Census) and four rural counties. Three stratified random samples were obtained: (a) 3,015 community residents age 18 and over, (b) an oversample of 906 community residents age 60 and older, and (c) 502 institutional residents from the same geographic area. The oversample of older adults was included to permit detailed examination of the prevalence and incidence of psychiatric disorders in later life. The analyses reported in this chapter are restricted to data from community-dwelling ECA respondents (both core community and elderly oversample).

At each ECA site, three interviews were obtained: a first personal interview; a telephone survey, conducted 6 months after the first interview; and a second personal interview, administered 1 year after the first interview. The telephone interview was brief and focused on health service use and changes in demographic states. Information about psychiatric disorders was obtained only in the personal interviews. The data reported here are from both personal interviews—social factors were generally measured at the first interview and psychiatric status was assessed at the second interview. The sample size for these analyses is 2,956, which represents the number of respondents who provided complete data at both test dates. Attrition between test dates is due to respondent refusals (10% of original respondents), mortality (5%), and relocation from the survey tracking range (4%).

Post-stratification weights were calculated to (a) adjust for attrition related to respondent age, gender, race, and urban/rural residence; (b) adjust for probability of selection within households of different sizes; and (c) down-weight the elderly oversample to their proportion in the population. All analyses are based on weighted data. Detailed descriptions of the sampling, data collection, and weighting procedures are available elsewhere (Blazer et al., 1985; Eaton & Kessler, 1985).

Measures

Major Depression.   The measure of major depression was based on information collected using Version III of the Diagnostic Interview Schedule (DIS). The history, characteristics, and validity of the DIS are described by Robins, Helzer, Croughan, & Ratcliff (1981). Briefly, the DIS is a highly structured interview designed for use by lay interviewers and generates computer-based diagnoses according to DSM-III criteria (American Psychiatric Association, 1980). The DIS elicits the elements needed for a DSM-III diagnosis: presence of symptoms; their severity, frequency, and concurrence; age at onset; and time of most recent symptoms. Structured probes are used to determine whether each symptom was due to physical illness, the effects of alcohol or drugs, or was of psychogenic origin. Only the latter are used in the computer diagnosis of psychiatric disorder. The DIS/DSM-III disorder examined here is major depressive episode (henceforth, often referred to simply as *depression*). To preserve the temporal differentiation of risk factors and disease outcome as firmly as possible, analysis is restricted to depression with onset within the 6 months prior to the second interview.

Demographic Characteristics.   Standard demographic variables examined include age, gender, race, and urban versus rural residence. Age was retained in continuous form in the main effects model; in tests of interaction, age was divided into three categories: age 18–39, age 40–64, and age 65 and older. Gender, race, and place of residence are dummy variables, with women, Blacks, and urban residents coded as 1. Time-1 measures were used for the demographic characteristics.

Life Course Achievements.   Education was measured as years of schooling (range = 0–21). Income was measured using 16 categories ranging from $1,999 and under to $50,000 and over. Information was collected for both personal and household income; personal income is used in these analyses. Marital status was coded as a set of dummy variables representing: married, widowed, never married, and divorced/separated. In these analyses, divorced/separated is the omitted category. Time-1 measures were used for these social factors. Additional analyses were performed to determine whether changes in marital status between the first and second interviews were related to the onset of depression. The number of respondents reporting changes in marital status was too small to permit stable estimates of this effect.

Physical health was measured in terms of the number of chronic illnesses (potential range = 0–12; observed range = 0–7; because of skewness, this variable was recoded as 0, 1, 2, 3, 4, 5 or more). Other health indicators, including self-rated health and number of physical symptoms, were examined.

Those measures were less powerful predictors of onset of depression than number of chronic illnesses. Physical health was measured as number of chronic illnesses at the Time-1 interview.

Stressful life events were measured using a checklist of 20 events that include family events, health events, work events, and other types of changes. For each event reported, respondents were asked whether the event was positive or negative, was important or unimportant, and was expected or unexpected. The measure used in these analyses was number of negative events reported by respondents (potential range = 0–20; observed range = 0–9; because of skewness, this variable was recoded as 0, 1, 2, 3, 4 or more). The time frame for reports of events was the past year. Because of this time frame, the life events measure is the one predictor based on Time-2 interviews. More detailed information about the life events inventory used in this study is available in Hughes, Blazer, and George (1988) and Hughes, George, and Blazer (1988).

Social Support. The Duke ECA interview schedule includes scales measuring four dimensions of social support: size of the social network, amount of interaction with the social network, instrumental assistance received from the support network, and subjective perceptions of the adequacy and quality of social support. Only the subjective social support measure is included in these analyses (potential range = 9–27; observed range = 10–25). This scale exhibits excellent internal consistency in this sample (α = .89). The Time-1 measure of subjective social support was used in these analyses. Exploratory analyses indicated that the other dimensions of social support were less powerful predictors of onset of depression than the measure of subjective social support—a finding reported in other studies (e.g., Kessler & McLeod, 1985; Krause, 1987c; Wethington & Kessler, 1986). Where multiple indicators of a given construct were available (as was the case for physical health as well as social support), some pruning of indicators was needed to preclude multicollinearity.

Analysis Strategies

Both main and interaction effects are examined using logistic regression. Logistic regression is the technique of choice because the dependent variable is dichotomous and badly skewed. Antilogged coefficients are presented in the form of odds ratios, because of their ease of interpretation. When interpreting odds ratios, 1.0 represents lack of a relationship between the independent and dependent variables. Odds ratios greater than 1 indicate positive relationships between independent variables and the dependent variable. Odds ratios of less than 1 represent negative relationships between predictors and the outcome. In line with our interest in the degree to which social factors differ across age groups, all possible interactions between age and other risk factors were examined. Other possible interactions were not examined with the exception of that between life events and subjective social support. Although findings are inconsistent, many investigators have hypothesized and/or observed an interaction between stress and social support such that social support is especially important for persons experiencing high levels of stress (e.g., Gore, 1978; House, 1981; Turner, 1981; Wethington & Kessler, 1986). Given the importance of this relationship in the literature, it was advisable to examine it in the context of this study.

Results

Age Differences in Depression and Risk Factors. The prevalence of DIS/DSM-III major depression differed substantially across age groups (Table 5.1). Because of the time frame used, these are incident cases, with onset during the last 6 months. Rates of 6-month major depression at Time 2 were 2.14%, 2.09%, and .69% for the young, middle-aged, and older age groups, respectively. This age difference is statistically significant, although the only significant contrast is between the oldest group versus the young and middle-aged groups.

Most of the risk factors were significantly associated with age also. Successive age groups, from youngest to oldest, exhibited increased proportions of women and decreased proportions of Blacks and urban residents. Marital status was related to age in predictable ways. Middle-aged adults were the most likely to be married, older adults were the most likely to be widowed, and young adults were the most likely to have never married. Differences in the proportions of divorced and separated respondents, however, were small and nonsignificant across age groups. Education and income also were related to age in predictable ways. Average levels of education decreased across age groups. Reflecting differences in employment status, middle-aged adults had the highest incomes and older respondents had the lowest incomes on average.

Physical health was strongly related to age, with rates of chronic illness increasing substantially across successively older age groups. Stressful life events

TABLE 5.1
Prevalence (in percent) of Major Depression,
by Age Group, Duke ECA Sample[a]

Age	Prevalence of Depression
18–39	2.14
40–64	2.09
65 +	.69

[a]Time frame for prevalence is last 6 months, as ascertained at Time-2 interview. Thus, these are incident cases with onset within the previous 6 months.

TABLE 5.2
Logistic Regression Analysis of Onset of Major Depression

Independent Variable	Odds Ratio
Age	.96**
Gender (Female = 1)	1.36**
Race (Black = 1)	1.04
Place of residence (Urban = 1)	1.29*
Married	.98
Widowed	1.01
Never married	1.03
Education	.98
Income	.99
Physical illness	1.13*
Stressful life events	1.16**
Subjective social support	.93**

*$p \leq .05$; **$p \leq .01$.

were significantly related to age with larger numbers of events reported by young adults than by either middle-aged or older adults. Finally, subjective social support was unrelated to age. The majority of all age groups reported perceptions of adequate and high quality social support.

Main Effects Model.   The first logistic regression model estimates the main effects of the risk factors on major depression (Table 5.2). Six of the 10 independent variables were statistically significant predictors of major depression. As expected given the bivariate distribution, age was negatively related to major depression. Women and urban residents were at statistically greater risk of depression than their male and rural counterparts. Physical illness and stressful life events were associated with higher risk of major depression. Subjective social support operated as a protective factor—respondents with high levels of perceived support were less likely to experience the onset of major depression. Race, marital status, education, and income were not statistically significant predictors of the onset of major depression.

Interactive Effects.   The stress-buffering effect of social support was not observed in this sample. It should be noted, however, that in logistic regression analyses the interaction terms test for differences in the *odds* of a risk factor across levels of another risk factor. In contrast, in ordinary least squares regression, interaction terms test differences in *probabilities* rather than odds. As Kessler (1983) pointed out, depending on whether odds or probabilities are examined, different conclusions may be reached about the presence of interaction. Indeed, when examined as probability differences, the interaction between negative life events and subjective social support was statistically significant. As

TABLE 5.3
Logistic Regression Analysis of Onset of Major Depression,
Within Age Groups

Independent Variable	18–39	40–64	65 +
Gender (Female = 1)	1.41**	1.02	1.09
Race (Black = 1)	1.13*	1.01	.98
Place of residence (Urban = 1)	1.34**	1.06	1.09
Married	.98	.96	.92**
Widowed	a	1.00	1.01
Never married	1.02	1.14*	1.16*
Education	.94**	.97	.97
Income	.99	.99	.98
Physical illness	1.17**	1.06	1.04
Stressful life events	1.19**	1.21**	1.14*
Subjective social support	.92**	.94*	.94*

^aToo few widows in youngest age group to permit stable estimate.
*$p \leq .05$; **$p \leq .01$.

expected, life events increased the probability of major depression more among respondents with low levels of subjective support than among those with high levels of subjective support (see also, Landerman, George, Campbell, & Blazer, 1989).

The major interactions of interest are those between age and other risk factors for major depression. Two kinds of analyses were used to detect and interpret these interactions. First, interaction terms were added to the main effects model shown in Table 5.2. Seven statistically significant interaction terms were observed. Second, separate logistic regression analyses were performed for the three age groups (see Table 5.3). These equations provide more interpretable information regarding the differential effects of risk factors across age groups.

Table 5.3 illustrates the different effects of risk factors across age groups. The three demographic variables—gender, race, and urban versus rural residence—are statistically significant predictors of major depression only for respondents age 39 and younger. Two categories of marital status interact with age. Being married has a significant protective effect only for older respondents. Having never married is significantly related to major depression only among middle-aged and older respondents. Education and physical illness are significantly related to risk of major depression only among young adults. Note that stressful life events increase the risk for major depression and subjective social support protects against depression among all three age groups. Income is not a significant predictor of major depression for any of the age groups. These results suggest that age plays a substantial role in moderating the effects of social factors on major depression.

STUDY 2: AGE, SOCIAL FACTORS, AND RECOVERY FROM MAJOR DEPRESSION[1]

Review of extant literature reveals increasing interest in the outcome of depressive illness. A small, but growing number of studies address this issue. Studies of the natural history and/or long-term outcome of major depression yield inconsistent results. These inconsistencies may be due in large part to methodological factors, including different definitions of recovery and relapse, different data collection methods, and sample diversity (e.g., community vs. clinical samples, variations in proportions of subjects with concurrent physical and/or psychiatric illness). Despite these inconsistencies, these studies cumulatively suggest that (a) a significant proportion of persons with major depression have not recovered within a year or longer of onset (12%–67% in previous studies; Keller & Shapiro, 1981; Keller et al., 1984; Keller, Shapiro, Lavori, & Wolfe, 1982a; Murphy, 1983; Murphy, Woodruff, Herjanic, & Super, 1974; Rounsaville, Prusoff, & Padian, 1980; Wesner & Winokur, 1988) and (b) a significant minority of people who recover from an index episode will experience a new episode within a year to 16 months (20%–38% in previous studies) (Keller & Shapiro, 1981; Keller, Lavori, Rice, Coryell, & Hirschfeld, 1986; Keller, Shapiro, Lavori, & Wolfe, 1982b; Rounsaville et al., 1980).

Only limited information is available concerning the predictors of recovery from major depression. The types of predictors examined in one or more previous studies include clinical features of the index episode (e.g., Coryell, Lavori, Endicott, Keller, & VanEerdewegh, 1984; Kivela & Pahkala, 1989; Mann, Jenkins, & Belsey, 1981; Murphy, 1983), patients' social characteristics (e.g., Baldwin & Jolley, 1986); life events during the interval between baseline and followup assessments (e.g., Murphy, 1983); and the availability of supportive interpersonal relationships (Henderson, 1984; Henderson & Moran, 1983). At this point, no consistent predictors of recovery have been identified.

The relationship between age and outcome of major depression is particularly relevant to the purposes at hand. Two studies examined illness course and outcome among older adult samples. Murphy (1983) reports that only 33% of a sample of 124 depressed patients age 65 and older had recovered 1 year later. Baldwin and Jolley (1986) studied a sample of 100 patients age 65 and older who were depressed at baseline and followed them from 42 to 104 months. They reported that 58% of the sample recovered and remained well throughout the follow-up period; 15% recovered and then experienced new depressive episodes. These figures are within the range observed in age-heterogeneous samples, so it is difficult to determine whether age itself is associated with poor outcome. Four other studies compared younger and older depressed patients.

---

[1]The study described here summarizes research results that already have been published (George et al., 1989).

Mann et al. (1981) and Keller et al. (1986) reported that older patients were more likely to have chronic, unremitting episodes of depression than their younger peers. Wesner and Winokur (1988) also reported worse outcomes for older patients but attribute that to increased physical health problems. In contrast, Cole (1983) reported no age differences in likelihood of or time to recovery. Thus, at this point, it seems safe only to conclude that older depressed patients do no better in outcome than younger patients. In addition, we lack knowledge about the extent to which predictors of recovery from major depression are equally salient across age groups.

In this study, 20 clinical and social factors are examined as potential predictors of recovery from depressive illness in a clinical sample: gender, age, marital status, family history of suicide, family history of mental disorder, level of depressive symptoms at index episode, duration of depressive episode, history of previous depressive illness, concurrent dysthymia, mild cognitive impairment, concurrent alcohol abuse/dependence, concurrent generalized anxiety disorder, negative life events, positive life events, four dimensions of social support, and length of time between baseline and follow-up assessments. Subjects consist of 150 middle-aged and older depressed inpatients who were administered baseline interviews during their index hospitalization and were reinterviewed 6–32 months later. Results are examined in terms of the main effects of these predictors on recovery from depressive illness and the extent to which age interacts with other predictors of recovery.

Sample

The sample was drawn from psychiatric inpatients participating in the Duke University Center for the Study of Depression in Later Life, a multidisciplinary research program designed to contrast the phenomenology of depression in middle age (35–50 years) and later life (age 60 and older). All patients were first screened for significant depressive symptoms. This involved a check of patients' charts for psychiatric diagnoses and administration of the Center for Epidemiologic Studies Depression Scale (CES-D) (Radloff, 1977). Those patients with a diagnosis of affective disorder and/or a CES-D score of 16 or greater were enrolled in the research program. A score of 16 or more on the CES-D has been shown to be indicative of clinically significant depression (Radloff, 1977).

After a patient "passed" one or both of the screening criteria, a clinical psychologist administered the Duke Depression Evaluation Schedule (DDES) (a composite interview schedule). Diagnostic information was obtained using several sections of the Diagnostic Interview Schedule (DIS) (Robins et al., 1981), including the sections on major depression, mania, alcohol abuse/dependence, generalized anxiety disorder, and the Mini-Mental State Exam (MMSE)

(Folstein, Folstein, & McHugh, 1975). We enriched the DIS depression section by adding items on sleep problems and items to distinguish both major
depression with and without melancholia, and depression with and without
psychotic features. DDES and screening data were reviewed by a diagnostic
team and consensus DSM-III diagnoses were assigned to all participants. These
consensus diagnoses have been compared with diagnoses derived from interviews using the Schedule for Affective Disorders and Schizophrenia (SADS).
Clinicians administering the SADS interviews were blind to the DDES, the
screening data, and to the consensus diagnoses based on those data. Comparisons of consensus and SADS diagnoses indicate high concordance for the diagnosis of major depression (K = .83) and acceptable concordance for the distinction between major depression with and without melancholia (K = .61).

Follow-up interviews were conducted by telephone after 6–32 months. The
follow-up interview schedule included the CES-D, other questions about depressive symptoms and symptom episodes, questions about use of medications and
health services, and measures of social functioning. Of the 200 patients contacted, 177 participated in the follow-up interview. Four respondents had died,
5 were not competent to report reliable data, and 14 refused to participate.
Of the 177 participating subjects, 150 received a consensus diagnosis of major
depressive episode with (n = 56) or without (n = 94) melancholia at baseline.
These 150 subjects comprise the sample used in these analyses. Compatible
with the research design, these 150 subjects are in two age groups: age 35–50
(n = 77) and age 60 and older (n = 73).

Measures

Outcome of Depression. The dependent variable is outcome of depression as
measured by CES-D score at follow-up. For the multivariate analysis, CES-D
is used in continuous form (potential range = 0–60; observed range at follow-
up = 2–56). For descriptive analyses, the CES-D was split into two categories:
"recovered" (CES-D less than or equal to 15) and "nonrecovered" (CES-D
equal to or greater than 16). As noted previously, this cut-point is compatible
with that used in previous studies (Radloff, 1977).

Seven categories of independent variables were included in the analysis. All
the independent variables were measured at baseline (i.e., during the index
hospitalization).

Demographic Characteristics. Gender, age, and marital status were examined.
Gender and age group were coded as dummy variables with women and old
age (i.e., age 60 and older) coded 1. Marital status was coded as a set of dummy variables: married, widowed, divorced/separated, and never married. In
the multivariate analyses, married was the omitted category.

Psychiatric History.   Three measures were examined: presence versus absence of family history of suicide, family history of mental disorder, and previous episode(s) of major depression. All three measures were based on patients' self-reports in the DDES.

Clinical Features of Index Episode.   Three features were examined as potential predictors of recovery status: baseline CES-D score, duration of the depressive episode before the baseline interview, and presence versus absence of major depression with melancholia. Baseline CES-D scores were included as indicators of disease severity; in addition, in the multivariate analyses, we controlled on baseline CES-D scores to highlight the effects of other predictors on *changes* in levels of depressive symptoms. Duration of the episode was viewed as an indicator of chronicity and was assessed via patients' self-reports at the baseline interviews. Presence versus absence of melancholia was based on the consensus diagnoses described earlier.

Psychiatric Comorbidity.   To determine whether coexisting psychiatric conditions decreased the likelihood of recovery, we examined presence versus absence of three other DSM-III diagnoses: dysthymia, alcohol abuse and/or dependence, and generalized anxiety disorder. These diagnoses were based on responses to the DIS sections included in the DDES. We also examined presence versus absence of mild cognitive impairment, based on responses to the Mini-Mental State Exam. (No respondents exhibited severe cognitive impairment on the MMSE.)

Life Events.   The DDES included the same life-events checklist used in the Duke ECA Project and described earlier. Respondents were asked about the occurrence of life events in the past year. For each item reported, respondents also were asked to rate the event as positive or negative, as important or unimportant, and as expected or unexpected. For the purposes of these analyses, two measures of life events were examined: number of positive events (coded as none or one vs. two or more) and number of unexpected, important, negative events (coded as none vs. one or more). These measures permitted us to determine whether positive experiences promote recovery and whether stressful life events predict poorer outcome.

Social Support.   The Duke Social Support Index (Landerman et al., 1989) was used to generate information about four dimensions of social support. Size of network is measured by four items, including an indication of complexity. Amount of social interaction is a four-item index, measuring the frequency of the respondent's interactions with members of the support network. Instrumental support is a 13-item index, tapping tangible services that the respondent receives from network members. Examples of the tangible services included are help when sick; financial assistance; help with housework, home repairs, and meals; transportation; gifts; and advice about problems. Subjective social support is a nine-item scale, described earlier for the ECA sample. Internal consistency in this sample remains excellent (α = .87). Each of the four social support dimensions was categorized as impaired (code of 1 assigned to bottom fifth of the scale) versus unimpaired. Note that the first three measures tap relatively objective facets of social support, whereas the fourth dimension is a purely subjective evaluation.

Time to Follow-Up. It is important to note that all of the independent variables were measured at baseline, 6–32 months before assessment of recovery status. Because of the wide variation in the intervals between the two interviews, time to follow-up was included as a control variable in the multivariate analyses, and was examined as a potential correlate of recovery status.

Analysis Strategies

First, contingency table analysis was used to examine the bivariate relationships between the independent variables and outcome (recovered vs. nonrecovered). Subsequently, multiple regression was used to examine the effects of the independent variables on outcome levels of depressive symptoms with the effects of other predictors statistically controlled. In the regression analyses, follow-up CES-D score (in continuous form) was the dependent variable. Hierarchical regression was used to enter the baseline CES-D score (also in continuous form) as the first predictor examined; the other independent variables were entered in a subsequent step. This procedure, known as residualized change analysis, estimates the effects of the independent variables on changes in depressive symptoms between test dates. Finally, potential interactions among the independent variables were examined.

Results

Bivariate Relationships Between the Independent Variables and Recovery. Overall, 48% of the sample had recovered from their index episodes of depression at the follow-up interview (Table 5.4). Participants in the oldest age group were slightly less likely to have recovered than those in the younger age group, but that difference was not statistically significant.

Only a few of the independent variables were significantly related to outcome of depression. Among the demographic variables, only marital status was significantly related to recovery status. Unexpectedly, the married were significantly less likely to have recovered than respondents in other marital states. None of the measures of psychiatric history were significantly related to re-

TABLE 5.4
Recovery Status (in percent) at Follow-Up Interview

	Recovered	Not Recovered
Total sample	48	52
Age 35–50	50	50
Age 60 +	46	54

covery. Of the three clinical features of the index episode, patients with baseline CES-D scores of 16 or more and patients diagnosed as having major depression with melancholia were less likely to have recovered. Two of the four measures of psychiatric comorbidity were significantly related to outcome status: Persons with a diagnosis of dysthymia, as well as those with a diagnosis of generalized anxiety disorder, were less likely to have recovered. Neither measure of life events was significantly related to outcome. Two of the social support measures were significantly associated with recovery status: Patients who were impaired in social interaction and subjective social support at baseline were less likely to have recovered. Length of time to follow-up was unrelated to recovery.

Residualized Change Analysis. Table 5.5 presents the results of the residualized change analysis. Two regression models are presented. Model 1 presents the main effects model; Model 2 presents the results for the regression equation including significant interaction terms. The independent variables included in Table 5.5 also merit brief comment. Regression models including all of the independent variables described earlier were estimated initially. Subsequently, most of the independent variables that did not significantly predict outcome CES-D score were deleted from the models. Both age and gender were retained in the models, however, because the main effects for any variables in the interaction terms must be estimated.

The results for Model 1 indicate that higher baseline CES-D scores, being married, a baseline diagnosis of dysthymia, and impaired subjective social support are significant predictors of higher numbers of CES-D symptoms at follow-up. These relationships are in the same directions as those observed in the bivariate analyses. Several predictors that were significantly related to outcome in the bivariate analyses, however, were reduced to nonsignificance in the regression analysis (e.g., major depression with melancholia, generalized anxiety disorder, social interaction). In addition, one predictor was significant in the regression analysis that was not significant in the bivariate analyses: social network. Unexpectedly, however, impaired social network at baseline was associated with lower numbers of depressive symptoms at follow-up. Overall, the main effects model explains 31% of the variance in follow-up CES-D scores; this explanatory power is highly significant.

TABLE 5.5
Residualized Change Analysis of Recovery From Depression

Independent Variable	Model 1		Model 2	
	b	B	b	B
Baseline CES-D Score	0.32	0.26**	0.32	0.25**
Gender (Female = 1)	2.44	0.07	5.40	0.16*
Age (60 or older = 1)	0.98	0.03	2.50	0.08
Widowed	-8.43	-0.14*	-7.29	-0.12
Divorced/separated	-7.23	-0.14*	-8.70	-0.17*
Never married	-10.66	-0.13*	-10.47	-0.13*
Dysthymia	5.98	0.18*	5.65	0.17*
Unexpected, important negative events	-0.04	-0.00	0.65	0.02
Social network (high score = impaired)	-7.86	-0.24**	-6.46	-0.20**
Subjective social support (high score = impaired)	8.88	-0.20*	21.94	0.49***
Age by subjective social support	—	—	-14.04	-0.16*
Gender by subjective social support	—	—	-15.90	-0.28*
Intercept	6.12		3.09	
R^2	0.31***		0.37***	

$*p \leq .05; **p \leq .01; ***p \leq .0001.$
Source: George, Blazer, Hughes, and Fowler (1989, p. 482).

Model 2 is nearly identical to Model 1 in terms of the main effects of the independent variables. Note, however, that gender does not emerge as a significant predictor of depressive symptoms at follow-up until the significant interaction terms are added to the model. Inclusion of the interaction terms also increases the explained variance of the the model to 37%. Before interpreting the significant interaction terms, it should be noted that we also tested the stress buffering hypothesis for all four dimensions of social support. In no case was the interaction between life events and social support statistically significant.

As Model 2 indicates, two significant interactions were identified. The effects of subjective support were conditional on both age and gender. Interpretation of the interaction terms is facilitated by Table 5.6, which provides mean CES-D follow-up scores for study participants cross-classified by age and subjective support and by gender and subjective support. The mean CES-D outcome score for middle-aged patients with impaired subjective support is twice as high as the means for middle-aged patients with unimpaired subjective social support, and for older patients regardless of baseline levels of subjective social support. In addition, subjective social support is more strongly related to CES-D symptom levels at follow-up for men than for women. Thus, although perceptions of inadequate social support generally predict higher levels of depression at follow-up, they are especially potent predictors of outcome for middle-aged patients and for men.

TABLE 5.6
Comparisons of Mean CES-D Scores for Age and Gender Groups
by Subjective Social Support

Subgroup	Mean CES-D Score at Follow-Up
Middle-aged, impaired subjective social support	36.11
Middle-aged, unimpaired subjective social support	16.69
Old, impaired subjective social support	16.40
Old, unimpaired subjective social support	17.03
Men, impaired subjective social support	39.30
Men, unimpaired subjective social support	13.02
Women, impaired subjective social support	26.08
Women, unimpaired subjective social support	19.54

Source: George et al. (1989, p. 483).

DISCUSSION AND IMPLICATIONS FOR FUTURE RESEARCH

Before synthesizing results of these two studies and discussing their implications for future research, the relative strengths and limitations of the two studies should be noted. With regard to the study of social factors and the onset of major depression, major strengths include data from a representative community population, information about a broad range of social factors that may be relevant to the onset of depression, and use of a prospective research design to examine illness onset. Two major limitations also merit mention. First, because of the epidemiologic nature of the ECA data, little information is available about the clinical features of the depressive episodes observed among study participants and about family history of psychiatric disorder. Thus, it is possible that the dependent variable is heterogeneous in ways that cannot be described or taken into account with the data available. Second, the ECA data, like several other epidemiologic surveys (e.g., Blazer & Williams, 1980; Gurland, 1976; Gurland, Dean, Cross, & Golden, 1980), reveal a rather paradoxical pattern with regard to the depression data: Older adults exhibit considerably lower rates of major depression as measured diagnostically, but they also exhibit rates of depressive symptoms that are equal to—and, in some cases, larger than—those reported by younger and middle-aged adults (Blazer, Hughes, & George, 1987). This pattern has yet to be explained and may well be important for conclusions about the role of age in the onset of depression.

The study of recovery from depression also has both strengths and weaknesses. On the positive side, results of that study are based on a relatively large clinical sample in which the diagnosis of depression at baseline was carefully performed. In addition, the database permitted simultaneous examination of several categories of variables potentially affecting illness course and outcome. Another clear advantage is the prospective nature of the research design, in which predictors of depressive outcome were ascertained prior to and independent of follow-up status. This study also had at least three weaknesses, however. First, all study participants were recruited as inpatients at a single treatment facility. In addition, rather narrow inclusion criteria were used in defining the sample. Thus, generalization of our findings is necessarily restricted. Second, although careful diagnostic procedures were implemented during baseline assessments, follow-up status was based solely on a 20-item screening scale. Although the CES-D is a widely used instrument, with documented psychometric properties, it is clearly not comparable to a diagnostic evaluation. Third, results are based on a single follow-up interview that varied in time since baseline assessment. Our results suggested that the length of this interval was not related to follow-up CES-D scores. Nonetheless, use of a single follow-up, as compared to multiple follow-ups obtained at standardized intervals, precludes a fully dynamic view of illness course and outcome. We now have instituted multiple follow-up interviews at defined intervals, and plan to examine illness course in more complex ways in future analyses.

The results of these studies suggest that age plays a significant and more complex role in the onset and outcome of depressive illness than has been previously recognized. The importance of age is not found primarily in its main effects. In the study of onset of depression, age had a significant and negative main effect, but its role as a moderator of other predictors of illness onset was more impressive. In the study of recovery from depression, age did not have a main effect, but had a statistically significant and substantively large interaction with subjective social support. Results from both studies suggest that potential interactions of age with other predictors of onset and outcome of depression should be examined in future research.

A note of caution is prudent at this point. Although age was observed to moderate the effects of one or more predictors in both studies, we cannot know whether those interactions represent the effects of age or cohort. Both studies were prospective; nonetheless, they represent short-term observations of illness onset and recovery. Clearly, we cannot determine whether the age effects observed are due to developmental aspects of the aging process or differences across cohorts.

The nature of the interactions of age with social factors also merit comment. The social factors with which age interacted in our studies are those suggested by previous research as potentially relevant predictors of onset and/or outcome of depression. The age interactions observed generally suggested that those social factors are more powerful predictors of illness onset and recovery among younger (or middle-aged) than older adults. Specifically, gender, race, urban versus rural residence, education, and physical illness all were significant predictors of onset of depression only for younger respondents. Only marital status—

both being married and having never married—was a stronger predictor of illness onset for older than younger adults. Only one age interaction was observed with respect to recovery from depression, but it was substantial in magnitude. Subjective social support was a significant predictor of recovery for middle-aged but not older respondents. One possible explanation for these age differences is that certain social factors have different meanings or salience at different ages or stages of life. For example, physical illness may be more predictive of depression among younger adults because it is more unexpected at younger ages. Similarly, marital status may be unrelated to depression at younger ages because it is both common and normatively acceptable for young adults to have not yet established families of procreation. But issues of prevalence and normativeness cannot explain why demographic characteristics—specifically, gender, race, urban residence, and education—are related to onset of depression for younger but not middle-aged or older adults. It also is not clear why subjective social support is a significant predictor of recovery from depression for middle-aged but not older adults.

These findings suggest the need to identify predictors of onset and outcome of depression that are unique to older adults—or are at least more important for older than younger adults. It is apparently not sufficient to simply adopt theoretical perspectives developed on samples of younger adults (or on samples of adults of all ages), even though some predictors are important for all age groups (e.g., life events and subjective social support for the onset of depression). Two lines of effort appear particularly promising for identifying such predictors. First, models of the onset and outcome of depression in later life could be infused with increased theoretical creativity. Rather than simply adopting models developed on younger adults, creative thought should be given to the unique characteristics of later life (and/or current older cohorts) that may be related to onset of and recovery from depression. Second, the field is ripe for empirically grounded observational and qualitative studies of depression in later life. Such studies hold considerable promise for generating hypotheses concerning the unique facets of depression in later life.

Although not directly related to the role of age in the onset and outcome of depression, one additional issue raised by the results of the two studies merits further examination in future studies. Our study of the onset of depression suggested that marital status is associated with decreased likelihood of depression among middle-aged and older adults. In contrast, the study of recovery from depression suggested that being married is associated with decreased likelihood of recovery from depression among middle-aged and older adults. Similarly, smaller rather than larger social network size was related to recovery from major depression. These somewhat contradictory results are puzzling and intriguing. It is likely that the two samples are associated with different quality marriages and/or social networks. That is, it may be that the majority of marriages in a random community sample are of high quality and, hence, protective with regard to the onset of depression. In contrast, the marriages of depressed patients may be more likely to be of poor quality. Another possibility is that marriage is a resource with regard to onset of depression, but a liability with regard to recovery from depression for reasons not yet specified or understood. At any rate, the effects of marriage, and perhaps interpersonal relationships more generally, should be carefully examined in future studies of both onset of and recovery from depression.

In summary, from both research and clinical perspectives, better understanding of the onset, course, and outcome of depressive illness (and other psychiatric disorders) is needed. Additional effort is needed to identify the social factors that affect onset, course, duration, and outcome of illness. These results suggest that age may moderate the effects of multiple social factors and that there is still much to be learned about the role that age plays in the onset of and recovery from major depression.

ACKNOWLEDGMENT

Support for preparation of this paper was provided by two grants (MH35386 and MH40159) from the National Institute of Mental Health.

REFERENCES

American Psychiatric Association. (1980). *Diagnostic and statistical manual of mental disorders* (3rd ed.). Washington, DC: Author.

American Psychiatric Association. (1987). *Diagnostic and statistical manual of mental disorders* (rev. 3rd ed.). Washington, DC: Author.

Baldwin, R. C., & Jolley, D. J. (1986). The prognosis of depression in old age. *British Journal of Psychiatry, 149*, 574–583.

Blazer, D. G., George, L. K., Landerman, R., Pennybacker, M., Melville, M. L., Woodbury, M. A., Manton, K. G., Jordan, K., & Locke, B. Z. (1985). Psychiatric disorders: A rural/urban comparison. *Archives of General Psychiatry, 42*, 651–656.

Blazer, D. G., Hughes, D. C., & George, L. K. (1987). The epidemiology of depression in an elderly community population. *The Gerontologist, 27*, 281–287.

Blazer, D. G., & Williams, C. G. (1980). The epidemiology of dysphoria and depression in an elderly population. *American Journal of Psychiatry, 137*, 439–442.

Brown, G. W., & Harris, T. (1978). *Social origins of depression.* London: Tavistock.

Burks, N., & Martin, B. (1985). Everyday problems and life change events: Ongoing versus acute sources of stress. *Journal of Human Stress, 11*, 27–35.

Cole, M. G. (1983). Age, age of onset, and course of primary depression in the elderly. *Canadian Journal of Psychiatry, 28*, 102–104.

Coryell, W., Lavori, P., Endicott, J., Keller, M., & VanEerdewegh, M. (1984). Outcome in schizoaffective, psychotic, and nonpsychotic depression. *Archives of General Psychiatry, 41*, 787–791.

Cronkite, R. C., & Moos, R. H. (1984). The role of predisposing and moderating factors in the stress-illness relationship. *Journal of Health and Social Behavior, 25,* 372–393.

DeLongis, A., Coyne, J., Dakof, G., Folkman, S., & Lazarus, R. S. (1982). Relationship of daily hassles, uplifts, and major life events to health status. *Health Psychology, 1,* 110–136.

Dimond, M., Lund, D. A., & Caserta, M. S. (1987). The role of social support in the first two years of bereavement in an elderly sample. *The Gerontologist, 27,* 599–604.

Dohrenwend, B. S. (1973). Life events as stressors: A methodological inquiry. *Journal of Health and Social Behavior, 14,* 167–175.

Dressler, W. W. (1985). Extended family relationships, social support, and mental health in a southern black community. *Journal of Health and Social Behavior, 26,* 39–48.

Eaton, W. W., & Kessler, L. C. (Eds.). (1985). *Epidemiologic field methods in psychiatry: The NIMH epidemiologic catchment area program.* New York: Academic Press.

Folstein, M. F., Folstein, S. E., & McHugh, P. R. (1975). "Mini-mental state": A practical method for grading the cognitive state of patients for the clinician. *Journal of Psychiatry Research, 12,* 189–198.

George, L. K. (1989). Social and economic factors. In E. W. Busse & D. G. Blazer (Eds.), *Geriatric psychiatry* (pp. 203–234). Washington, DC: American Psychiatric Association.

George, L. K., Blazer, D. G., Hughes, D. C., & Fowler, N. (1989). Social support and the outcome of major depression. *British Journal of Psychiatry, 154,* 478–485.

Gore, S. (1978). The effect of social support in moderating the health consequences of unemployment. *Journal of Health and Social Behavior, 19,* 157–165.

Gurland, B. J. (1976). The comparative frequency of depression in various adult age groups. *Journal of Gerontology, 31,* 283–292.

Gurland, B. J., Dean, L., Cross, P., & Golden, R. (1980). The epidemiology of depression and dementia in the elderly: The use of multiple indicators of these conditions. In J. O. Cole & J. E. Barrett (Eds.), *Psychopathology of the aged* (pp. 127–141). New York: Raven Press.

Henderson, S. (1981). Social relationships, adversity and neurosis: An analysis of prospective observations. *British Journal of Psychiatry, 138,* 391–398.

Henderson, A. S. (1984). Interpreting the evidence of social support. *Social Psychiatry, 19,* 49–52.

Henderson, A. S., & Moran, P. A. P. (1983). Social relationships during the onset and remission of neurotic symptoms: A prospective community study. *British Journal of Psychiatry, 143,* 467–471.

Holahan, C. K., & Holahan, C. J. (1987). Self-efficacy, social support, and depression in aging: A longitudinal analysis. *Journal of Gerontology, 42,* 65–68.

Holahan, C. K., Holahan, C. J., & Belk, S. S. (1984). Adjustment in aging: The role of life stress, hassles, and self-efficacy. *Health Psychology, 3,* 315–328.

House, J. S. (1981). *Work stress and social support.* Reading, MA: Addison-Wesley.

Hughes, D. C., Blazer, D. G., & George, L. K. (1988). Age differences in life events: A multivariate controlled analysis. *International Journal of Aging and Human Development, 27,* 207–220.

Hughes, D. C., George, L. K., & Blazer, D. G. (1988). Age differences in life event qualities: Multivariate controlled analyses. *Journal of Community Psychology, 16,* 161–174.

Kanner, A. D., Coyne, J. C., Schaefer, C., & Lazarus, R. S. (1981). Comparisons of two modes of stress measurement: Daily hassles and uplifts versus life events. *Journal of Behavioral Medicine, 4,* 1–39.

Kaplan, H. B., Robins, C., & Martin, S. S. (1983). Antecedents of psychological distress in young adults: Self-rejection, deprivation of social support, and life events. *Journal of Health and Social Behavior, 24,* 230–243.

Keller, M. B., & Shapiro, R. W. (1981). Major depressive disorder: Initial results from a one-year prospective naturalistic followup study. *Journal of Nervous and Mental Disease, 169,* 761–767.

Keller, M. B., Shapiro, R. W., Lavori, P. W., & Wolfe, N. (1982a). Recovery in major depressive disorder. *Archives of General Psychiatry, 39,* 905–910.

Keller, M. B., Shapiro, R. W., Lavori, P. W., & Wolfe, N. (1982b). Relapse in major depressive disorder. *Archives of General Psychiatry, 39*, 911–915.

Keller, M. B., Klerman, G. L., Lavori, P. W., Coryell, W., Endicott, J., & Taylor, J. (1984). Long-term outcome of episodes of major depression. *Journal of the American Medical Association, 252*, 798–792.

Keller, M. B., Lavori, P. W., Rice, J., Coryell, W., & Hirschfeld, R. M. A. (1986). The persistent risk of chronicity in recurrent episodes of nonbipolar major depressive disorder: A prospective followup. *American Journal of Psychiatry, 143*, 24–28.

Kessler, R. C. (1979). Stress, social status, and psychological distress. *Journal of Health and Social Behavior, 20*, 259–272.

Kessler, R. C. (1983). Methodological issues in the study of psychosocial stress. In H. B. Kaplan (Ed.), *Psychosocial stress: Trends in theory and research* (pp. 267–341). New York: Academic Press.

Kessler, R. C., & McLeod, J. D. (1985). Social support and mental health in community samples. In S. Cohen & S. L. Syme (Eds.), *Social support and health* (pp. 219–240). New York: Academic Press.

Kivela, S. L., & Pahkala, K. (1989). The prognosis of depression in old age. *International Psychogeriatrics, 1*, 119–133.

Krause, N. (1986). Social support, stress and well-being among older adults. *Journal of Gerontology, 41*, 617–622.

Krause, N. (1987a). Chronic financial strain, social support, and depressive symptoms among older adults. *Psychology and Aging, 2*, 185–192.

Krause, N. (1987b). Life stress, social support, and self-esteem in an elderly population. *Psychology and Aging, 2*, 301–308.

Krause, N. (1987c). Chronic strain, locus of control, and distress in older adults. *Psychology and Aging, 2*, 375–382.

Landerman, R., George, L. K., Campbell, R. T., & Blazer, D. G. (1989). Alternative models of the stress buffering hypothesis. *American Journal of Community Psychology, 17*, 625–642.

Lin, N., & Ensel, W. M. (1984). Depression-mobility and its social etiology: The role of life events and social support. *Journal of Health and Social Behavior, 25*, 176–188.

Lin, N., Simeone, R. S., Ensel, W. M., Kuo, W. (1979). Social support, stressful life events, and illness: A model and an empirical test. *Journal of Health and Social Behavior, 20*, 108–119.

Lin, N., Woelfel, M. W., & Light, S. C. (1985). The buffering effect of social support subsequent to an important life event. *Journal of Health and Social Behavior, 26*, 247–263.

Mann, A. H., Jenkins, R., & Belsey, E. (1981). The twelve-month outcome of patients with neurotic illness in general practice. *Psychological Medicine, 11*, 535–550.

Monroe, S. M. (1983). Major and minor life events as predictors of psychological distress: Further issues and findings. *Journal of Behavioral Medicine, 6*, 189–205.

Murphy, E. (1983). The prognosis of depression in old age. *British Journal of Psychiatry, 142*, 111–119.

Murphy, G. E., Woodruff, R. A., Herjanic, M., & Super, G. (1974). Variability of the clinical course of primary affective disorder. *Archives of General Psychiatry, 30*, 757–761.

Norris, F. H., & Murrell, S. A. (1984). Protective function of resources related to life events, global stress, and depression in older adults. *Journal of Health and Social Behavior, 25*, 424–437.

Radloff, L. S. (1977). The CES-D Scale: A self-report depression scale for research in the general population. *Applied Psychological Measurement, 1*, 385–401.

Robins, L. N., Helzer, J. E., Croughan, J., & Ratcliff, K. (1981). National Institute of Mental Health Diagnostic Interview Schedule: Its history, characteristics, and validity. *Archives of General Psychiatry, 38*, 381–389.

Rounsaville, B. J., Prusoff, B. A., & Padian, N. (1980). The course of nonbipolar, primary major depression. *Journal of Nervous and Mental Disease, 168*, 406–411.

Turner, R. J. (1981). Experienced social support as a contingency in emotional well-being. *Journal of Health and Social Behavior, 22*, 357–367.

Wesner, R. B., & Winokur, G. (1988). An archival study of depression before and after age 55. *Journal of Geriatric Psychiatry and Neurology, 1*, 220–225.

Wethington, E., & Kessler, R. C. (1986). Perceived support, received support, and adjustment to stressful life events. *Journal of Health and Social Behavior, 27*, 78–89.

Wheaton, B. (1983). Stress, personal coping resources, and psychiatric symptoms: An investigation of interactive models. *Journal of Health and Social Behavior, 24*, 208–229.

Williams, A. W., Ware, J. E., & Donald, C. A. (1981). A model of mental health, life events, and social supports applicable to general populations. *Journal of Health and Social Behavior, 22*, 324–336.

Zarski, J. J. (1984). Hassles and health: A replication. *Health Psychology, 3*, 243–251.

Cohort Experiences, Support Versatility, Depressive Traits, and Theory

Stanley A. Murrell
University of Louisville

First, a comment that is a response both to George's chapter and more generally to all of the contributions in this volume. It seems a natural and useful evolution for a field of study to progress through cycles of research. The first cycle perhaps entails the throwing of a wide net to encompass a broad range of variables but within a certain conceptual perspective. The first cycle serves to both reveal more clearly the complexity of relationships and to rule out those hypotheses, relationships, and variables that appear to be unimportant to the phenomena being studied. The comprehensiveness of this cycle eventually yields a better "big picture" of the phenomena and a new perspective gradually emerges that changes the roles of different variables.

A conceptual shift seems to be occurring now in the study of stress and resources. What have been seen up to now primarily as control variables are now seen as independent variables having greater substantive value and deserving of new attention. In this volume, George suggested this for age, House for socioeconomic variables, James for race, and Berkman's findings suggested this for gender.

What is the nature of the conceptual shift? Surely, it is too early in the shift to see this very clearly. Most explicit in the contributions to this volume is the need to better explicate the context. Each of these "demographic" variables illuminates the personal experience context of aging and health. A much less explicit shift may be the recognition of the need to *extend* the context by studying the phenomena over a longer *temporal* field. Embedded in age, gender, race, and social class are experiences that are life long, extending back many years before the researcher arrives to take a measurement "snapshot."

* * *

In her chapter, George raises a number of intriguing questions with important implications for the future study of social support and depression in older adults. Her emphasis on the need for theory seems particularly important for this area of study at this time in its history.

COHORT EXPERIENCES

George interprets her findings of age by social factor interactions as suggesting that there is a need to identify predictors of depression that are unique to older adults, or at least of greater importance for them. She suggests developing new theory that considers the specific qualities of older age, or of current older cohorts, as integral to that theory, and she suggests more fine-grain studies of depression as experienced by older persons.

Some would no doubt object to the idea of age-specific theories. One concern might be of a possible stigmatizing effect—any admission that older adults are different might be used against them. Others may translate "age-specific" as suggesting rigid, uni-directional stages, and feel that this would be going backward, theoretically. Others may react on the basis that chronological age is considered by some as a weak explanatory variable. I discuss this latter point at greater length here.

Over the past 40 years, various researchers have offered the opinion that chronological age itself is not useful as a *causal* variable. More recently, Maddox and Campbell (1985) discussed the need to combine social structural variables and personal variables in the same research. They pointed out that "cohort" is a higher order concept than chronological age because it incorporated the interaction of person (or individual experiences) and environment (or socialization effects); that is, cohort has greater potential as an explanatory variable than chronological age. And, George carefully acknowledges that her findings of age differences may well reflect cohort differences rather than maturational differences.

In her onset study, George characterizes subjective social support as a protective factor—those who perceive themselves to have strong support are less likely to have an onset of major depression. In that same logistic regression analysis (see Table 5.2) age has the same sign and essentially the same value as social support. Thus, could *age* also be a *protective factor*? This would be a conceptual shift from our prevailing view of age as a disadvantage. *Or*, could this particular cohort have had experiences that were protective? This is developed further here.

Eysenck (1983) has argued that exposure to chronic stress inoculates the organism to the effects of future stress on health. Or, prior experiences facilitate adaptation to current stress. In our longitudinal studies of older adults, we have generally found life events to have weak and temporary effects on physical and mental health, even events as significant as bereavement, suggesting the possibility that greater experience with changes by virtue of living longer may give older adults an adaptational advantage over younger persons (e.g., Murrell & Himmelfarb, 1989; Murrell, Himmelfarb, & Phifer, 1988; Norris & Murrell, 1987, 1988).

As a specific example, Norris and Murrell (1988) found that, with prestress symptoms controlled, older adults who had had prior experience in floods had fewer symptoms after a new flood than those without prior flood experience. Having survived an earlier flood, these older adults were less anxious in the current flood.

From a historical perspective, persons who are in their early 80s today experienced the great depression in their early 20s, or as they were entering the job market and beginning careers. They then experienced World War II when they were in their 30s as parents with young families. Did these historical events, occuring at these family developmental stages, have socialization effects and inoculation effects that make current-day 80-year-olds less at risk for depression than other 80-year-olds? Past and future 80-year-olds? *Or*, does having lived for 80 years itself give most persons experience with changes that then serve to inoculate them against the effects of current changes?

The general point here is that *cohort* as a variable can serve as a surrogate for experiences, both societal and personal, that have potential explanatory and theoretical value for studying health in older adults. In the same sense that George recommends studying age not as a control but as a substantive variable, cohort can be viewed not as a methodological problem but as a substantive opportunity.

To adopt inclusion of cohort experiences as a general practice means, of course, that our research would need to collect measures with a longer temporal perspective, which would also make it more difficult, complex, and expensive.

SOCIAL SUPPORT VERSATILITY

The summary sentence for this next topic might be: "Social support works in mysterious ways." In her onset study, George found that marital status interacted with age: Being married reduced the risk of onset only for the older respondents; having never married was not related to depression among the younger respondents. Yet, in her recovery study, George found that being married made recovery less likely for the middle-aged and older respondents. Subjective social support was positively related to recovery for the middle-aged, yet social network size was inversely related to recovery, seemingly counterintuitive. *And yet*, these results are not surprising! Many other studies have *also* yielded social support findings that are unexpected and puzzling!

In his review that has since become the classic in the social support area, Cassel (1976), an epidemiologist, concluded that social support was a protective factor for health in the face of stress. This paper helped start the current interest in social support as a buffer of stress effects on health. In his review, Cassel cited a number of animal studies in which animals were more vulnerable to health effects of stress if they were isolated, or if they were exposed in the company of unfamiliar animals. Clearly, we do not know the *perceived* social support of these mice and goats! The most evident social support dimension in these animal studies is familiarity. Familiarity currently is not in vogue as a social support dimension. Furthermore, in the human studies that Cassel reviewed, social disorganization, familiarity, and predictability were more apparent dimensions than social embeddedness or perceived support.

The point here is not that only those dimensions identified by Cassel are the correct dimensions, but that there are many different dimensions of social support that may be important. Nor is the point to add familiarity as yet another dimension of social support. My fear is that the proliferation of social support dimensions will leave the field with many bits and pieces, rather than accumulated knowledge. What is needed, it seems to me, is more conceptual work, in the manner of Sheldon Cohen and his colleagues (e.g., Cohen & Wills, 1985), to bring greater cohesion and deeper understanding to the field of social support.

Also, what we measure may not be the social support dimension that we think it is! In a recent study by Kaniasty, Norris, and Murrell (1990), a measure of what we thought was perceived support was taken on an early wave as part of a longitudinal study *before* the respondents were exposed to a flood disaster. (We like to call this our devine intervention design.) Items on this scale asked how much help was expected from various sources during an emergency. This scale was administered before the floods. Generally, the respondents expected to have rather strong support. *After* the flood, we measured the amount of support the respondents had actually received during the disaster, using the same items with minor word changes, essentially asking how much support they had indeed received during the flood emergency from different sources. We also had additional measures of perceived support on subsequent waves after the flood (15 to 18 months following the flood).

We found that the flood victims received less support than they had expected. However, receiving less support than they expected did not change their post-flood perceptions of potential support. That is, the reality of support during the flood did not influence their social support expectations *after* their flood experience. Their illusion of high levels of support was not dashed by experience! Rather than measuring perceived social support, we may have been measuring some type of support *optimism trait*! Obviously, there are several possible explanations for this; the point is that respondent experience may not coincide with our labels.

George found social support to have direct effects on both onset and recovery from depression, and a support by events interaction with onset (depending on the analysis), but no buffer effect on recovery. Social support has often been found to have direct effects on physical and mental health, but not totally consistently; findings for the buffer effect have also been inconsistent in both health areas (e.g., Berkman, 1986; Blazer, 1982; Cohen, 1988; Cohen, Teresi, & Holmes, 1985; Cutrona, Russell, & Rose, 1986; Schaefer, Coyne, & Lazarus, 1981). We have found social support to be generally stable over time (Norris & Murrell, 1987), and social support often is related to subsequent negative life events, with strong support making negative events less likely (Murrell & Norris, 1991).

Thus, social support can apparently have multiple effects, and these effects can vary with dimension, dependent measure, sample, event experiences, and statistical procedure. Fran Norris and I have done a study of persons who experienced a death of spouse during a longitudinal project (Norris & Murrell, 1990). Pre-death social embeddedness, essentially a measure of the strength of social network prior to the death of spouse, had direct effects on depression following the death (an average of 9 months following the death); embeddedness did not have a direct effect on physical health. Perceived support did not have significant effects. Also, strong social embeddedness reduced the subsequent global stress experienced following the death. And, a strong social network during bereavement made the coping activity of developing new interests more likely, which further reduced depressive symptoms. Thus, social embeddedness had direct, moderating, and mediating effects on depression. It seemed to serve both deterrent and coping functions.

This complexity makes social support a difficult variable to study. But it also suggests that as a resource social support is versatile and effective.

One approach has been to view this complexity as a methodological problem rather than as reflecting the nature of the phenomena. The preferred solution seems to be rather reductionistic, defining more and more dimensions of social support. Indeed there are benefits to greater specification, and this seems to be the trend in the life events literature as well (e.g., Thoits, 1987). The problem with this is that it may give rise to more and more unconnected findings. My suggestion is to include different support dimensions in the same study, then compare the strength and patterns of their respective effects.

As something of a footnote here, Phifer and Murrell (1986) found that the strongest predictor of onset of depressive symptoms in our older adult sample was an interaction of social support and health, strong support combined with good physical health made an increase in symptoms above the cutpoint less likely. Given George's finding that health was related to onset only in the younger sample, it would be interesting to see whether this health by support interaction would vary in different age groups.

DEPRESSIVE TRAITS

Over 10 years ago, Warheit (1979) noted the intraperson consistency across time in depressive symptom checklist scores and suggested that this reflected a depressive trait. Most of us have known colleagues, patients, and even family members with a depressive trait.

In our studies, we have consistently found the strongest single predictor of depressive symptoms to be prior depressive status (i.e., level of depression on the preceding wave). In George's recovery study, baseline CES-D was not the strongest predictor, but it was among the strongest. I would urge that prior health status be considered as a substantive independent variable, as a surrogate of the respondent's personal history with the dependent variable.

This consistency of depressive symptoms is typically underplayed in most studies, since some other independent variable was usually the purpose of the study. The exception to this is the work of Paul Costa and his colleagues (e.g., Costa et al., 1986). A methodological implication of this consistency is that if your intention is to predict *change* in depressive symptoms, you will often have little change to predict. The public health implication of this consistency is that depressive symptoms are reliable identifiers of persons at risk for future high levels of depressive symptoms.

THEORY

In closing, I want to second George's call for "an infusion of increased theoretical creativity" not only for depression in later life, but for gerontology in general. As a pertinent example, I would recommend a conceptual framework developed by Pilisuk (1982) that considers the mechanisms, including physiological chains, that may underly the relationship of social support to physical illness. The field and this conference have been rich in data, but not in conceptualization. In this era of the microchip, we can continue to extend our list of predictors without necessarily deepening our understanding of the phenomena.

Also, George suggests more qualitative, and as I interpret it, richer studies of the experience of depression in older adults. Almost in passing, she suggests this type of information as a basis for generating hypotheses, or theory, not exclusively as providing increased knowledge for itself. I strongly agree, and I would add that older adults who have experienced life changes and successfully adapted are survivors and as such are important sources for theories of *protective* health behaviors.

REFERENCES

Berkman, L. (1986). Social networks, support, and health: Taking the next step forward. *American Journal of Epidemiology, 123*, 559–562.

Blazer, D. (1982). Social support and mortality in an elderly community population. *American Journal of Epidemiology, 115*, 684–694.

Cassel, J. (1976). The contribution of the social environment to host resistance. *American Journal of Epidemiology, 104*, 107–123.

Cohen, C., Teresi, J., & Holmes, D. (1985). Social networks, stress, and physical health: A longitudinal study of an inner-city elderly population. *Journal of Gerontology, 40*, 478–486.

Cohen, S. (1988). Psychosocial models of the role of social support in the etiology of physical disease. *Health Psychology, 3*, 269–297.

Cohen, S., & Wills, T. (1985). Stress, social support, and the buffering hypothesis. *Psychological Bulletin, 98*, 310–357.

Costa, P., McCrae, R., Zonderman, A., Barbano, H., Lebowitz, B., & Larson, D. (1986). Cross-sectional studies of personality in a national sample: 2. Stability in neuroticism, extraversion, and openness. *Psychology and Aging, 1*, 144–149.

Cutrona, C., Russell, D., & Rose, J. (1986). Social support and adaptation to stress by the elderly. *Psychology and Aging, 1*, 47–54.

Eysenck, H. (1983). Stress, disease and personality: the "inoculation" effect. In C. Cooper (Ed.), *Stress research* (pp. 121–146). New York: Wiley.

Kaniasty, K., Norris, F., & Murrell, S. (1990). Received and perceived social support following a natural disaster. *Journal of Applied Social Psychology, 20*, 85–114.

Maddox, G., & Campbell, R. (1985). Scope, concepts, and methods in the study of aging. In R. Binstock & E. Shanas (Eds.), *Handbook of aging and the social sciences* (pp. 3–31). New York: Van Nostrand Reinhold Company.

Murrell, S., & Himmelfarb, S. (1989). Effects of attachment bereavement on subsequent depressive symtoms in older adults. *Psychology and Aging, 4*, 166–172.

Murrell, S., Himmelfarb, S., & Phifer, J. (1988). Effects of bereavement/loss and pre-event status on subsequent physical health in older adults. *International Journal of Aging and Development, 27*, 89–107.

Murrell, S., & Norris, F. (1991). Differential social support and life event stress as contributors to the social class–distress relationship. *Psychology and Aging, 6*, 223–231.

Norris, F., & Murrell, S. (1987). Transitory impact of life-event stress on psychological symptoms in older adults. *Journal of Health and Social Behavior, 28*, 197–211.

Norris, F., & Murrell, S. (1988). Prior experience as a moderator of disaster impact on anxiety symptoms in older adults. *American Journal of Community Psychology, 16*, 665–683.

Norris, F., & Murrell, S. (1990). Social support, life events, and stress as modifiers of adjustment to bereavement by older adults. *Psychology and Aging, 5*, 429–436.

Phifer, J., & Murrell, S. (1986). Etiologic factors in the onset of depressive symptoms in older adults. *Journal of Abnormal Psychology, 95*, 282–291.

Pilisuk, M. (1982). Delivery of social support: The social inoculation. *American Journal of Orthopsychiatry, 52*, 20–31.

Schaefer, C., Coyne, J., & Lazarus, R. (1981). Health related functions of social support. *Journal of Behavioral Medicine, 4*, 381–406.

Thoits, P. (1987). Gender and marital status in control and distress: common stress versus unique stress explanations. *Journal of Health and Social Behavior, 28*, 7–22.

Warheit, G. (1979). Life events, coping, stress and depressive symptomatology. *American Journal of Psychiatry, 136*, 502–507.

Statistical and Causal Interaction in the Diagnosis and Outcome of Depression

Carmi Schooler
National Institute of Mental Health

The research reported by George in chapter 5 answers important questions about how social-structural factors interact with age to affect the onset and outcome of depression. It does so by carrying out sensible analyses of state-of-the-art interview data gathered from a sophisticatedly selected representative sample of individuals in the community. It also uses similarly sophisticated methods to examine the course of illness of a reasonably representative sample of patients hospitalized for the treatment of major depression.

George's results point to several interesting conclusions: Age may moderate the effects of various social factors on depression—being female, urban, Black, poorly educated, and physically ill increases the chances of becoming depressed at younger, but not older ages. On the other hand, being married, which is not related to depression among young adults, is associated with a decreased likelihood of depression among middle-aged and older adults. Marital status has an intriguingly different relationship to recovery from depression among older adults. In this population, being married, and also having a large social network decreased the chance of recovering after hospitalization.

Although ultimately convincing, George's analyses and findings raise important methodological and substantive issues. In this chapter, I begin by discussing a few methodological qualms I have about the specific analyses carried out. These qualms reflect more general concerns about what I see as problematic in much of the research linking psychiatric epidemiology to social factors. In doing so, I focus on a methodological issue—the importance of considering interactions in epidemiological research—that I have discussed previously in the context of cross-cultural research on schizophrenia (Schooler, 1989), but which is equally relevant to research on depression, social structure, and the

169

life course. I show that interactions are important both in terms of defining the problems considered and in arriving at appropriate conclusions. Switching to a more directly substantive issue, I then suggest some explanations for the apparently paradoxical findings that George presents. Based on my own somewhat similar findings on schizophrenics (Schooler & Parkel, 1966), these tentative explanations, which imply the existence of causal interactions, raise questions about how social factors may interact with the course and nature of mental illness.

METHODOLOGICAL CONCERNS

My methodological concerns revolve around three issues: (a) overdependence on subjective measures where more objective ones could have been used, (b) the loss of information due to discarding multiple indicators, and (c) the nature of the test for interactions. In regard to the first issue my qualm is that the measure of social support that George uses has been somewhat arbitrarily limited to the respondent's subjective estimate. The reason given—the fact that other more objective measures of social support were less powerful predictors of the onset of depression—is just what makes me uneasy. One of the symptoms of depressive affect is to believe that one is unloved, unwanted, and uncared for. Thus, subjective estimates of social support may well be affected by the illness, and part of the high correlation between depression and reports of low social support may be the result of a causal path from depression to the report. Such a path would clearly not be as substantively interesting as one in the opposite direction—that is, from the absence of social support to depression. At a minimum, if a subjective measure of social support is used, a reciprocal effects model should be estimated.

My second concern is the use to which multiple indicators are put. As someone with a bias toward confirmatory factor analysis and linear structural equation modeling, I am made uneasy by the statement that "Where multiple indicators of a given construct are available (as was the case for physical health as well as social support), some pruning of indicators was needed to preclude multicollinearity." It is just such a multiplicity of indicators of an underlying construct that makes it possible for confirmatory factor analysis to take into account the effects of measurement error (Joreskog & van Thillo, 1972). Because differences in the amount of measurement error in independent variables strongly affect their regression weights, such differences become important when we are trying to decide the degree to which different social background and individual history variables affect the likelihood of depression.

My third concern has to do with the likelihood of finding interactions being affected by the fact that the search for interactions is carried out in terms of whether the odds that a risk factor will be linked to a diagnosis of depression change across levels of another risk factor. As I understand it, in such an analysis interactions are found to exist only when the ratios change. Thus, if the shift of the odds between two levels of Variable A on one level of Variable B is from 2% to 4%, and the shift between the two levels of Variable A on the second level of Variable B is from 20% to 40%, no interaction would be found. For those of us accustomed to using analyses of variance or ordinary least squares to estimate interactions, this result would seem surprising. However, George's approach is probably appropriate if one is trying to assess how much a given variable affects the likelihood that an individual will fall into a given diagnostic category. Assessing the probability that individuals with certain characteristics will fall into the diagnostic category of major depression is the purpose of this part of George's analysis. From my perspective, however, it is the relationship between the presence of interactions and the use of diagnostic categories in epidemiological research that is the basis of the most general methodological issue I want to raise.

Interactions, Diagnoses, and Epidemiology

In assessing the relationship between social factors and the onset of depression, George uses the DIS/DSM-III criteria for whether a given individual qualifies as a case of major depressive illness. These criteria were developed by the Epidemiologic Catchment Area (ECA) investigators as a way of establishing, through the use of the Diagnostic Interview Schedule (DIS), that a respondent should be diagnosed as fitting the Major Depression Diagnoses established by the American Psychiatric Association Diagnosis and Statistical Manual of Mental Disorders (DSM-III, 1980). In order to meet these criteria, a respondent to the DIS had to report being sad and/or anhedonic for at least 2 weeks and also to report having at least four out of a set of eight other symptoms. Essentially what we have here is an interaction effect. Thus, a diagnosis of depression cannot be made simply in terms of an individual's state on only one of these criteria (e.g., being very sad, or having more than four of the eight symptoms), but must be made on the basis of an interaction among the two. As I show later, the assumption that such an interaction is necessary for a diagnosis to be useful is essentially correct. Unfortunately, however, such assumptions are generally made without their validity being tested or their implications being fully understood.

The relevance of statistical interactions to the diagnostic process can best be understood if we first model the potential types of interactions that can occur in the relationships between predictors and outcomes. In order to describe such relationships in formal terms (see Table 1), let us assume we have a set

TABLE 1
Types of Relationships Between Predictors and Outcomes

Outcome (X) occurs	Nature of Model	Predictors		
		A	B	C
1. Only if A	Pathognomic (single-predictor)	necessary & sufficient	not nec.	not nec.
2. If either A and/or B and/or C	Cumulative–Multiple (alternative or additive)	suf.	suf.	suf.
3. Only if A and B	Interactive–Restrictive	nec.	nec.	not nec.
4. Only if A and either B and/or C*	Interactive–Alternative	nec.	nec. if no C	nec. if no B

*In a more general statement of the Interactive-Alternative Model, A, B, and C can be considered as alternative sets of phenomena: one from each set of which is necessary if an interaction is to occur (i.e., one from Group A, one from Group B and one from Group C).

of possible predictors (A, B, C) for an outcome X. Both predictors and outcomes can be events, psychological or physical symptoms, or diagnoses. Both predictors and outcomes can be linear or categorical. If predictors are linear, they can imply a threshold triggering level. Such a threshold, which assumes non-linearity of effect, can be seen as analogous to an interaction, in that the results of moving from one point in the scale to the next are a function of the position on the scale where the movement occurs. For example, the difference between having two or having three of the symptoms necessary for a DIS/DSM-III diagnosis of depression is less important than the difference between having three or having four of these symptoms because four is the threshold value that has to be passed for the diagnosis to be given.

The timing of a predictor may also be part of its definition (e.g., A at Time 1 may be defined as not equal to A at Time 2). In addition, the previous occurrence of a similar phenomenon may be part of the definition of a predictor (e.g., A [second occurrence] is not equal to A [first occurrence]). The inclusion in a definition of limitations that are based on time or on number of occurrences should, however, be grounded on firm empirical demonstrations that such limitations significantly improve predictive power. Predictions or diagnoses should be made at the earliest time possible. Thus, for example, the goal should be to distinguish those who will relapse from those who will not, as long before the relapse occurs as possible. It should also be remembered that for those trying to understand the implications of an event that occurs at a given time, including in the definition determining the meaning of that event the occurrence of a later event makes it impossible to be sure of the meaning of the earlier event when it occurs. Doing so is like including an outcome among the predictors in a regression analysis.

Table 1 describes four types of relationships between predictors and out-comes. Two are not interactive: Pathognomonic, the case where a particular predictor is both necessary and sufficient, and Cumulative–Multiple, where any member of a set of predictors, either by itself or when cumulated with other predictors of that set, would be sufficient to predict an outcome. Two are interactive: the Interactive–Restrictive case requires the co-occurrence of at least two particular predictors for an outcome to occur; the Interactive–Alternative one requires the co-occurrence of at least one predictor from each of two sets of phenomena.

Even if we disregard for a moment the concerns voiced by sociologists and psychologists about the appropriateness of the "medical model," a long-stand-ing question in the area of psychiatric epidemiology is whether emphasis should be placed on case identification and diagnosis or on describing the nature of the psychological functioning and psychiatric symptomatology of the popula-tion being studied. The case-finding approach, in which the occurrence of a particular illness is ascertained on the basis of pre-established diagnostic criteria or the judgment of a certified expert, is frequently seen as best suited for plan-ning medical services. In a sense however, even from the perspective of medi-cal planners, identifying a case is a less germane psychiatric problem than treat-ing dysfunctional symptoms. From a scientific point of view, limiting one's concern to sorting individuals into pre-ordained categories involves both the potential waste of a great deal of data and the acceptance of the assumption that the diagnostic system one is working with is correct and universally appli-cable, even though this assumption is particularly problematic in life course re-search. If psychiatric epidemiologists, instead of limiting themselves to ascertain-ing the number of cases in a population, analyze the past and present symptoms and levels of functioning of the individuals they sample, it becomes possible for them to validate their diagnostic criteria, to test alternate sets of criteria, and to assess the applicability of competing diagnostic approaches in different contexts.

A diagnosis is valid to the extent that it improves prediction of such out-comes as the course of symptomatology, the efficacy of different forms of treat-ment or the understanding of the nature of underlying causal mechanisms. Unless a particular symptom or event is pathognomonic for a given outcome (Model 1 in Table 1), a diagnosis is based on more than one symptom or event. It is in the examination of how such multiple symptoms and events predict a particular outcome that the focus on interactions takes on importance. *Only if there is a statistical interaction among the component symptoms* (i.e., Models 3 or 4 in Table 1) *does the establishment of a diagnosis (or syndrome) improve the ability of a set of symptoms to predict an outcome above what would be known by examining how much each separately adds* (i.e., Model 2 in Table 1) *to our knowledge of that outcome.* Thus, multisymptom-based diagnoses are scientifically advantageous only if they are based on an Interactive–Restrictive or Interaction–Alternative model of the relationship between predictors and outcomes.

A concern for interactions also has practical implications for the construction of questionnaires and other instruments for assessing psychiatric status. Such instruments have to be constructed in such a manner that they do not foreclose the possibility of testing for interactions among potentially relevant symptoms. In order to do this, they have to be in a format that encourages the recording of all potentially relevant symptoms, rather than the "expeditious" placing of the individual into one of a series of preordained diagnostic categories.

An example of how symptom ratings can be systematically examined for interactive effects can be found in a study by Kellam (1989). He investigated how teachers' ratings of students' maladaptive symptom-like behaviors (i.e., shyness, aggressiveness, immaturity, underachievement, concentration problems) in the first grade predict delinquency, substance abuse and psychiatric symptoms 10 years later. Using log linear modeling, he found that despite the intercorrelations among them, the individual scales work independently in predicting later outcomes—suggesting that the Cumulative–Multiple model applies. The major exception is that aggressiveness and shyness do not work independently but interact together in predicting later outcomes, indicating that the Interactive–Restrictive model is operating for these traits. Kellam viewed these results as implying that shy–aggressiveness, which resembles the DSM-III category of Undersocialized Conduct Disorder, is a valid syndrome. The logic he followed in coming to this conclusion essentially parallels that of this discussion.[1]

How might the view of the relationship between interaction and diagnoses that I am proposing affect the conclusions that can be drawn from George's study of depression? Given the approach I am suggesting, the emphasis on the DIS/DSM-III diagnosis of depression would be soft-pedaled in favor of a series of dimensional analyses that would test for the existence of the interactions underlying the hypothesized diagnosis. Latent class analysis might also be used to see whether certain symptoms significantly occur together, and whether these co-occurring symptoms are related to either background factors or prognosis.

One hint within George's data that the DIS/DSM-III diagnosis may not be completely appropriate is the puzzling finding that although the rates of diagnosed depression are considerably lower in older people than in younger ones, older people exhibit equally high, or higher, rates of depressive symptoms than younger individuals. One possible explanation of this finding is that certain symptoms have different meanings among older than among younger

---

[1]One difference in logic between our approaches is that Kellam is concerned that the occurrence of symptoms that make up a particular diagnosis be highly correlated. This is not necessarily important. For example, although the presence of fever may be necessary for the diagnosis of a particular disease, given all of the different causes of a fever, the occurrence of a fever is not necessarily very highly correlated with the occurrence of all of the other symptoms of that disease.

individuals. Thus, two frequently cited signs of depression—sleep disturbance and loss of interest in sex—may be less diagnostically meaningful among older than younger individuals. It is plausible that if such possibly false indicators of depression are not counted, the elderly would fail to show more "depressive" symptoms and their lower level of diagnosed depression would seem less paradoxical. On the other hand, the nature of depression may well be different in the elderly, so that different diagnostic patterns should be sought out.

In any case, we are dealing with issues of interactions, either among symptoms or between symptoms and individual characteristics such as age. Another example of such an interaction is the apparently greater effect of social factors on the diagnoses of depression in the younger than in the older respondents. Here too, however, we do not know if this is true for the various components of the diagnosis. Because the nature of the interaction among symptoms has not been systematically explored, the applicability of the DIS diagnostic procedure for depression to the elderly is in some question. Consequently, the implications of the interactions among the various social and personal background factors—especially aging—also remain in question.

Paradoxical Findings: Some Substantive Implications

Despite the length of my methodological digression, I remain impressed with the methodological sophistication of George's research. More to the point, I am convinced that the picture it portrays of social factors and the onset and outcome of depression is essentially correct. Such a conviction, however, forces me to accept the truth of its apparently paradoxical result that at least two variables (not being married and having relatively small social networks) that increase the likelihood of being diagnosed as depressed also increase the likelihood of recovery (see Table 2).

TABLE 2
Paradoxical Findings

Schizophrenia (Schooler & Parkel, 1966)	Conditions that increase the likelihood of Schizophrenia but decrease the pathology in a hospitalized chronic population
	History of mental illness in the family
	Low level of relationship with the opposite sex (not married men)
	Parental absence
Depression (George, chapter 5, this volume)	Variables that increase likelihood of onset of depression but also increase the likelihood of recovery
	Not being married
	Having a relatively small social network

Part of my willingness to accept such apparently paradoxical results is that I have found somewhat similar ones myself when studying schizophrenia. It is possible that the explanations that were developed for my findings with schizophrenics may also be applicable to depressives. I raise these possibilities despite my trepidation in moving from a subject I know something about—schizophrenia—to one in which I am definitely not expert—depression.

As noted in Table 2, in a study done in 1962 on the relationship of the overt behavior of chronic schizophrenics to their internal state and personal history (Schooler & Parkel, 1966), we found that a history of mental illness in the family, a low level of relationship with the opposite sex, and parental absence, all predictors of the occurrence of schizophrenia, also predicted relatively low levels of pathology among hospitalized patients. At the time, we explained these findings by hypothesizing the existence of a selective process in the determination of who was discharged from the hospital. Because this was the historical period during which deinstitutionalization was just beginning, it seemed plausible that those patients with interested spouses or parents would be more readily discharged. In a somewhat similar manner, those with a family history of mental illness would be relatively accepting of hospitalization and be less likely to have reasonable homes to go to and would consequently be likely to remain in the hospital, even if they were in relatively good psychological shape.

A somewhat similar explanation may also explain the findings about depression—if one assumes that depressives who are married or who have relatively large social networks would only be brought into the hospital when they are unresponsive to outpatient treatment. On the other hand, those who did not have such support systems before hospitalization may have benefited from the support the hospitalization supplies.

Another hypothesis, which may hold true for both schizophrenics and depressives, is that those who get sick in the presence of what generally seem to be prophylactic conditions may have a stronger predisposition (biological or psychological) toward the illness or a more intractable form of it. Whichever of these explanations proves true, we are dealing with interaction, but of a different sort than that involved in the problem of diagnosis. Here, the interaction involves the pattern of causal interrelationships of the patient's psychological functioning, illness, treatment, social situation, and background.

CONCLUSIONS

Using George's analyses and findings as a starting point, I have tried to demonstrate the importance of considering statistical and causal interactions in the study of the diagnosis and outcome of depression. Elsewhere (Schooler, 1989), I have similarly tried to show how the consideration of such interactions is important for the study of the diagnosis and etiology of schizophrenia. The importance of examining such interactions in psychiatric epidemiology transcends the investigation of these two major mental illnesses. Such an approach can help resolve some of the more general questions that have been raised in the sociological literature about the scientific legitimacy of the whole process of psychiatric diagnosis.

In their harsh attack on psychiatric diagnosis in general, and the DSM-III and DIS in particular, Mirowsky and Ross (1989) went so far as to "recommend eliminating diagnosis from research on the nature, causes, and consequences of mental, emotional, and behavioral problems" (p. 11). They arrive at this conclusion by arguing that "diagnosis treats attributes as entities; . . . reduces the signal but not the noise; and . . . collapses . . . structural relationships" (p.11). In invited comments on the Mirowsky and Ross paper, Klerman (1989), Swartz, Carroll, and Blazer (1989) and Tweed and George (1989) strongly defended psychiatric diagnostic procedures on the basis of these procedures' demonstrated importance for the advancement of knowledge about the biology, genetics, treatment, and prognosis of mental disorder. However, even these staunch and able defenders of the DSM-III and DIS diagnostic approaches agree that it is unfortunate that the hostile polemic style of the Mirowsky and Ross article may lead to the overlooking of some reasonable questions that it raises.

It is in the context of the question of whether psychiatric diagnosis merely represents a reification of measurement procedures, which both legitimate and are legitimated by the psychiatric profession, that I believe that the model proposed in Table 1 is heuristically useful. In particular, I believe that psychiatric diagnoses could be empirically validated if that model were used to examine how psychiatric symptoms and other relevant variables predict the "commonly agreed-upon external validators" of diagnoses that Klerman (1989) listed: "a) clinical course and outcome; b) response to treatment; c) findings from laboratory tests; d) family and genetic studies; and e) correlation with social-demographic, personality and life events" (p.29).

Based on what is already known, I strongly suspect that in terms of the major mental illnesses, the present diagnostic criteria will prove to be essentially correct. Nevertheless, as someone who has spent decades trying to deal with the high level of psychological and biological variance of those carrying schizophrenic diagnoses, I would not be surprised if the statistical interaction oriented approach to psychiatric diagnosis I am proposing would lead to meaningful changes in exactly how diagnostic boundries are drawn. However, as George's findings suggest is the case for depression, the search for such empirically validated diagnostic classifications may be complicated by a second type of interaction—the causal interaction of the nature and course of individuals' illnesses and treatment histories with their stage in the life course and position in the social system.

REFERENCES

American Psychiatric Association. (1980). *Diagnostic and Statistical Manual of Mental Disorders* (3rd ed., DSM-III). Washington DC: Author.

Joreskog, K. G., & van Thillo, M. (1972). *LISREL: A general computer program for estimating a linear structural equation system involving multiple indicators of unmeasured variables* (ETS Research Bulletin 72-56). Princeton, NJ: Educational Testing Services.

Kellam, S. G. (1989). Developmental epidemiological framework for family research on depression and aggression. In G. R. Patterson (Ed.). *Depression and aggression in family interaction* (pp. 11-48). Engelwood Cliffs, NJ: Lawrence Erlbaum Associates.

Klerman, G. L. (1989). Psychiatric diagnostic categories: Issues of validity and measurement. Invited comment on Mirowsky and Ross (1989). *Journal of Health & Social Behavior, 30,* 26-32.

Mirowsky, J., & Ross, C. (1989). Psychiatric diagnosis as reified measurement. *Journal of Health & Social Behavior, 30,* 11-15.

Schooler, C. (1989). A statistical interaction approach to problems in cross-cultural epidemiology. In E. K. Yeh, H. Rin, C. C. Yeh, & H. G. Hwu (Eds.), *Prevalence of mental disorders: Proceedings of International Symposium on Psychiatric Epidemiology* (pp. 339-357). Taiwan: Dept. of Health, the Executive Yuan, Republic of China.

Schooler, C., & Parkel, D. (1966). The overt behavior of chronic schizophrenics and its relationship to their internal state and personal history. *Psychiatry, 29;* 67-77.

Swartz, M., Carroll, B., & Blazer, D. (1989). In response to "Psychiatric diagnosis as reified measurement." Invited comment on Mirowsky and Ross. *Journal of Health & Social Behavior, 30,* 33-34.

Tweed, D. L., & George, L. K. (1989). A more balanced perspective on "Psychiatric diagnosis as reified measurement." Invited comment on Mirowsky and Ross. *Journal of Health & Social Behavior, 30,* 35-37.

6

Aging, Health Behaviors, and Health Outcomes: Some Concluding Comments

James S. House
University of Michigan

As the introduction by my colleague and co-organizer, Dan Blazer, suggests, what might be termed the *psychosocial epidemiology of health and aging* has grown remarkably over the past several decades. This conference was held at the end of a decade in which the growing enthusiasm of the 1940s–1970s for epidemiology, social science, and psychosocial epidemiology gave way to some increasing uneasiness or skepticism in many quarters, and an increased tendency to view psychosocial and biomedical approaches to the study of aging and health as inherently competitive. These recent trends reflect increasing resource scarcity, which subjects all endeavors to more questioning and more competition. They also reflect the increasing growth and maturity of the social epidemiology of both health and aging. As Dan Blazer suggested, we have learned a great deal over the past several decades. We are also at a point where we need to take stock and consider directions for the future.

The chapters and discussions presented here reflect this state of the field. They build upon the progress of prior decades, yet manifest a search for new directions and priorities. Without attempting to summarize the contents of the chapters or discussions, this conclusion suggests ways in which this volume both reflects the progress of the last several decades and suggests major issues and agendas for the future.

Current developments in both the psychosocial and biomedical study of health and aging must be viewed in historical perspective. In the two decades immediately following the end of World War II, what might be termed the *biomedical approach* to health and aging reached its zenith in many ways. The "germ theory" of disease and its associated doctrine of specific etiology led, via both vaccination and drug therapy, to the completion of the conquest of infectious diseases in the developed countries, and had a major impact on reducing mortality from such diseases in developing nations as well. The discovery of DNA and RNA promised new avenues for the intervention and control of genetically transmitted diseases and perhaps even for unlocking the long-sought "fountain of youth." With the introduction of Medicare in 1965, all older Americans were to be guaranteed equal access to the wonders of modern medicine. I entered graduate school that year, and soon after discovered a fledgling field of study of psychosocial factors in health, but it had as yet had no major impact on the dominant biomedical paradigm.

The biomedical approach to health and aging continues to be dominant today, and many biomedical scientists remain skeptical of psychosocial approaches, perhaps increasingly so as the competition for resources for both research and clinical practice intensifies. These realities should not, however, prevent recognition that the relative positions, and perhaps even trajectories, of the biomedical and psychosocial approaches to health and aging have changed dramatically in the last quarter century. During the 1960s and early 1970s the biomedical model did not deliver the gains in quantity and quality of life that had been expected and hoped for. The steady increase of life expectancy during the first half of this century was arrested for the first time beginning in the late 1950s. With the emergence of chronic diseases as the major causes of morbidity and disability, and our inability to really cure such diseases, even continued gains in life expectancy were ambivalently characterized as yielding "longer life but worsening health" (Verbrugge, 1984). The later 1970s and 1980s saw renewed gains in life expectancy, even for people at older ages, but the sources of this have been attributed as much to behavioral and psychosocial changes (e.g., changes in lifestyle such as not smoking, diet, and exercise) as to prophylactic and therapeutic medical or surgical interventions (Goldman & Cook, 1984). By the late 1970s, nonmedical factors were identified as the major determinants of mortality (DHEW, 1979). And the extent to which the years we are adding to life are healthful ones remains much in dispute (*Gerontologica Perspecta*, 1987).

The past quarter century has brought increasing identification of the role of specific psychosocial factors in the etiology of mortality, morbidity, and functional limitations from both physical and psychological disorders. The chapters by Kaplan, Satariano, and George build upon and reflect these trends. The Alameda County Study, major findings from which are reviewed by Kaplan, played a seminal role in establishing "lifestyle" variables (i.e., smoking, drinking, obesity, physical activity, and perhaps sleep patterns), as major risk factors for mortality. These data and those from other studies led to a series of Public Health Service reports on the risks of unhealthy life styles, and resultant changes in social policy and individual behavior that have dramatically altered patterns of smoking, drinking, eating, and physical activity in the general population, which in turn contributed to reductions in mortality, morbidity, and probably also disability (U.S. Surgeon General, 1964; DHEW, 1979; DHHS, 1988).

The Alameda County Study and other research have more recently established in varying degrees that social relationships and supports, chronic and acute stress, and personal efficacy and control are important predictors or risk factors for mortality and morbidity. More limited data indicate that changes in these factors can reduce mortality and morbidity, or improve the course of aging and chronic illness (cf. chapters by Kaplan, George, and Satariano and also House, Landis, & Umberson, 1988; Rodin, 1986; Rowe & Kahn, 1987). It is important to recognize that the social factors are important for both the etiology and the course of morbidity, and that the kind of evidence for their effects is increasingly similar to that for biomedical risk factors such as blood pressure or blood lipids. This evidence includes both large scale prospective epidemiological studies (among them the Framingham, Tecumseh, and Evans County studies that were the major sources of understanding of biomedical risk factors) and experimental laboratory or nonexperimental or field studies on both animals and humans.

In summary, the psychosocial approaches to health and aging have achieved a degree of scientific legitimacy and credibility in the last quarter century that few could have predicted in the 1960s. The biomedical model remains dominant, but with greater awareness of its limits and the need for complementary psychosocial approaches. This is a major achievement for psychosocial epidemiology and the social sciences. It is also the source of the challenge that now confronts us. Where do we go from here?

The chapters and discussions contained in this volume suggest that psychosocial approaches to health and aging must move increasingly in several directions. First, we need to continue and accelerate efforts to relate the study of psychosocial factors in aging and health to issues of both biological process and clinical and public practice, as is suggested especially in the comments of Blazer, Cohen, Ostfeld, and Schooler, and in Blazer's introduction to this conference and volume as well. Second, as the comments of Siegler especially suggest, we need to focus increasingly on morbidity and functional status as outcomes, and not just on mortality or life expectancy. Finally, we need to understand better the broader social context in which psychosocial factors affect aging and health, as suggested especially in the chapters by myself and colleagues and by James and colleagues, and in the comments of Maddox and Williams on these chapters and of Murrell on the George chapter. Because the first two issues have been extensively discussed in the chapters and comments and in the larger literature, and because of my perspective as a sociologist, I conclude with some comments on the need to focus more on the larger social context in which psychosocial factors relate to aging and health.

As Stanley Murrell puts it: "A conceptual shift seems to be occurring now in this field. What have been seen up to now primarily as control variables are now seen as independent variables having greater substantive value and deserving of new attention.'' And he refers specifically to age, race, gender, and socioeconomic status (SES). He and others are interested in these variables because they define the position of individuals in the social structures of society, especially its systems of social stratification, and hence, importantly define and determine the current, past, and future life conditions and experiences to which individuals are exposed (see also Pearlin, 1989). In varying degrees age, race, gender, and SES also determine or are related to significant aspects of the functioning and change of individuals as biological organisms. Thus, age, race, gender, and SES account for a great deal of the variation in health in our society. Understanding how and why this is so is critical to further progress in preventing or postponing the onset of mortality, morbidity, and functional limitations, and to improving health in an aging society.

Running through most of the chapters and comments is increased recognition that age is not just a chronological correlate or determinant of changes in health status. Rather age also represents a social and biological context which may both determine exposure to psychosocial as well as biological risk factors to health and also modify the impact of a wide range of risk factors on health. Further, age combines not only additively, but also interactively, with gender, race, and SES in predicting health. That is, race, gender, and SES differences in health vary substantially across age levels, or alternatively the relation of age to health varies by race, gender, and SES (and perhaps combinations thereof), although without better longitudinal data we cannot be sure whether these differences are due to aging of individuals or differences between cohorts.

Understanding the social meaning, contexts, and experiences associated with age, race, gender, and SES can improve future research, clinical practice, and health policy in aging and health, even with regard to psychosocial factors in aging and health. Williams argues eloquently in his discussion that health behaviors, social relationships and supports, chronic and acute stress, personal efficacy and control, and other social factors linked to health are themselves determined by the social conditions in which people live, which are stratified by age, race, gender, and SES. Understanding how these social stratification variables relate to health helps to identify high-risk populations and some of the more proximal psychosocial factors responsible for such risk. Hence, they can help us to better target clinical and public health interventions.

Equally or more importantly, however, they represent new targets for public health and perhaps even clinical interventions. That is, we can seek not only to modify directly the levels of health behaviors, stress, social relationships, supports, or personal efficacy and control that individuals experience, but we can also seek to alter the broader social conditions and contexts that bring about or reinforce these psychosocial risk factors. We can even seek to affect absolute and relative levels of socioeconomic status. Although gender, race, and age cannot, of course, be altered, we can attempt to alter the patterns of social opportunities and barriers associated with those immutable ascribed statuses. Some will argue that we cannot change such variables. But, in fact, all of these social conditions and contexts have been altered significantly in the past. And three or four decades ago, many were equally skeptical that we could reduce smoking, change diet and exercise patterns or fluoridate water supplies, yet we have.

Increased attention to those broader social factors in health will also help us to address problems in our current understanding of psychosocial factors in health. A number of papers and discussions note that we often fail to understand how various psychosocial risk factors (e.g., health behaviors, social relationships and supports, efficacy or control) relate to each other. Age, race, gender and SES importantly determine or modify the impacts of all of these variables. Hence, consideration of these broader social forces and contexts will force us to focus more on interrelationships among sets of psychosocial risk factors that are currently studied too much in isolation from each other.

In summary, we are at an important juncture in the study of psychosocial factors in aging and health. The relevance of multiple psychosocial variables to processes of aging and health is now undeniable. Yet we also need to understand better how these risk factors relate both to more microscopic biomedical factors and more macroscopic social factors in health and aging. It is only because we have come such a long way in this area in the past several decades, that we can now see that we still have far to go in the coming decades. The chapters and discussions in this conference and volume appropriately reflect the past progress, the current problems, and the future promise of efforts to understand the role of psychosocial factors in aging and health.

ACKNOWLEDGMENT

Preparation of this chapter has been partially supported by the National Institute of Aging (Grant #P01AG05561). I am indebted to Marie Klatt for preparing the manuscript.

REFERENCES

Gerontologica Perspecta. (1987). Issue on the compression of morbidity, *1*, 3–66.

Goldman, L., & Cook, E. F. (1984). The decline in ischemic heart disease: An analysis of the comparative effects of medical interventions and changes in lifestyle. *Annals of Internal Medicine, 101*, 825–836.

House, J. S., Landis, K., & Umberson, D. (1988). Social relationships and health. *Science, 241*, 540–545.

Pearlin, L. I. (1989). The sociological study of stress. *Journal of Health and Social Behavior, 30*, 241–256.

Rodin, J. (1986). Aging and health: Effects of the sense of control. *Science, 233*, 1271–1276.

Rowe, J. W., & Kahn, R. L. (1987). Human aging: Usual and successful. *Science, 237*, 143–149.

U. S. Department of Health, Education, and Welfare. (1979). *Healthy people: The Surgeon General's Report on Health Promotion and Disease Prevention.* Washington, DC: U. S. Government Printing Office.

U. S. Department of Health and Human Services. (1988). *Promoting health/preventing disease.* Washington, DC: U. S. Department of Health and Human Services.

U. S. Surgeon General's Advisory Committee on Smoking and Health. (1964). *Smoking and health.* Washington, DC: U. S. Public Health Service.

Verbrugge, L. M. (1984). Longer life but worsening health? Trends in health and mortality of middle-aged and older persons. *Milbank Memorial Fund Quarterly/Health and Society, 62*, 475–519.

Author Index

The page numbers listed below include text citation locations only. For complete bibliographical information, please see the reference sections at the end of each chapter.

Subject Index